The Necklace
of
Occasional Dreams

a woman's journal of living with her husband's cancer

Kathleen Winter

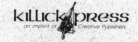

killick press
an imprint of Creative Publishers

St. John's, Newfoundland
1996

Grief was often the first lifeline uttered in a diary. . . . In bereavement the chief pain of the loss comes from the loss of self. An investment has been made in the loved one: spouse, child, parent, friend. The closer the love has been, the deeper the emotional investment. In order to survive and continue with one's own life, one has to withdraw the self that was entrusted to the other person. This is what grieving is all about.

Betty Jane Wylie
Reading Between the Lines: The Diaries of Women

The Necklace
of
Occasional Dreams

a woman's journal of living with her husband's cancer

Kathleen Winter

The publisher acknowledges the financial contribution of the *Department of Tourism and Culture, Government of Newfoundland and Labrador,* which has helped make this publication possible.

Appreciation is expressed to *The Canada Council* for publication assistance.

Photos, front and back covers, Manfreid Buchheit

∝ Printed on acid-free paper

Published by

KILLICK PRESS A CREATIVE PUBLISHERS IMPRINT
a division of 10366 Newfoundland Limited
a Robinson-Blackmore Printing & Publishing associated company
P.O. Box 8660, St. John's, Newfoundland A1B 3T7

Printed in Canada by:
ROBINSON-BLACKMORE PRINTING & PUBLISHING

Canadian Cataloguing in Publication Data

Winter, Kathleen

 The necklace of occasional dreams
 ISBN 1-895387-62-0

1. Cancer — Pateints — Family relationships.
2. Cancer — Patients — Newfoundland — Biography.
3. Wade, James — Health. I. Title.

RC280.L8W56   1995   362.1'9699424'0092 +   C95-950298-X

CONTENTS

Part I:
Do Handsome Princes
Eat Cinnamon Toast?

July 3, 1992

I want to start a notebook now before too much else happens. If this is to be a long haul then too much can be forgotten. I wish this was the book on wildflowers I was going to write, but it isn't. James was diagnosed June 8 with cancer of the lung. Now he has had two bronchoscopies, two biopsies, and a mediastinoscopy. The results of the last test will be ready, the surgeon says, on Monday. This is Friday.

The mediastinoscopy is what James had today. Dr. Gardiner said there was a small "risk." I did not say, "A small risk of what?" James asked Dr. Gardiner if he could eat after the operation, and Dr. Gardiner said he could probably eat his lunch.

At 11:30, three hours and fifteen minutes after the operation, which was said to take about an hour usually, I realized nobody was going to phone me and tell me anything. I did the usual round of busy signals and transfers and on holds that anybody else does when they call a hospital, and finally found from his room-mate Mike that James could not talk. "Can he hear?" I asked him. Yes. I said tell him I'll be there in a few minutes.

I took a taxi there. I walked along the corridor of 5 East preparing myself visually. The books I have read, and the doctors, describe a mediastinoscopy as a very small procedure —hardly an operation at all. I hadn't been prepared to hear Mike say that James couldn't talk.

When I went in I saw that they had hurt my husband. He was pale and disoriented. He could not get up. His face was swollen. He was wearing a hospital johnny suit, but it had fallen off his back. His neck had a fat oblong bandage puffing out, and his whole chest and shoulders were uncovered. His chest and shoulders were painted with a smeared brown substance, and two dark ribbons of dried blood were snaking from beneath the bandage and down over his back. He could hardly speak and kept drifting to sleep. I kissed him and stroked him. The pillow had plastic under the cover, and it wasn't thick enough. Jim's hand had an IV needle in it; the dripping bag of salt water hung beside him. I kissed him and stroked him until I had to get Esther from the day care where she goes part-time. Jim looks after her in the afternoons — I have a day job, and am wondering what is going to happen about that. I took today and yesterday off, but I can't take every day off and still keep the job.

I left him asleep and found the nursing station. I went in and said to two nurses, "Excuse me." They didn't turn around. I said to their backs, "I am James Wade's wife, and I was wondering if anyone is going to wash all the brown stuff off him" — They were looking at me by now — "and there's dried blood running down his back as well." The nurses smiled and were warm then. They said they would surely wash him — that they didn't do it right away because he was resting. Later on the phone Jim said two nurses came in and sponged him and told him they were doing it because his wife had expressed concern for him. That made me feel good. Later I went to the hospital again and he was so much better.

His face was pink again and he was washed. He was my Jimmy again.

July 5, 1992

Before James went into the hospital, I wanted to shoot a roll of film of us — James, Esther and me. but I never got around to it. I saw a picture one morning that I will never forget.

He was taking her to the day-care centre; they were walking hand in hand down the driveway. I was watching them through the living room window. They went down, the new maple leaves filling the air over their heads, sunshine falling in dapples on Esther's sun-hat, on J's browny-gold hair. Esther's sun-hat was new — white with a brim and red trim. I had put a blue corduroy pinafore dress on her, red tights and her new sneakers. Her legs were lovely and long. When they walked down the hill together I felt them precious and dear. James had just had his thirty-ninth birthday, and Esther had recently had her third. I told myself it didn't matter if there was no picture. Photographs don't always retain the whole love and tenderness of a moment, and memory, while it lives, is more sensitive to these things.

July 6, 1992

Esther cried in bed then said, "I'm crying because Daddy is sick." She spends a lot of time with her daddy when things are normal. This morning before we brushed our teeth, she was standing on the toilet the way she does so she can reach the sink, and I said give me a standing-up hug. She gave me a cuddly one and said, "Marry me! Marry me!" in a plaintive tone. I remembered her Beauty and the Beast cards, one of which has Beauty and the prince standing up, hugging. "I'm the Beast," Esther said. "Yes, I'll marry you, " I told her, hugging her. "Oh look — you're a handsome prince now!"

"Do handsome princes like cinnamon toast?" she asked me. "Yes," I said. "They love it. Do you want some now?" She said yes.

This evening when the surgeon and interns entered room 5107, James and I were lying in his bed under the sheets reading a magazine. They laughed and we did too. I got out of the bed and sat down. They told us Dr. Spurrell was right, it is cancer, and Dr. Gardiner thought surgery was really the only option, and with our permission it could proceed around the middle of this week, when he can get operating-room time. It looked like he wasn't going to elaborate on what type of cancer it was, so I asked. "It's called large cell cancer," he said, and I knew James felt relieved. I was glad of the books Nancy had sent, so we knew something about it. After they left, James danced around the hospital room grinning, singing, "I've got cancer," to the tune of "Frere Jacques" — a tune we had used for one of our own baby songs about Esther. We both felt a great temporary relief, which came partly from being told something conclusive after this torture of waiting.

July 14, 1992

Things are not very good. The operation was not a success. Dr. Gardiner took me aside and told me that the cancer is more extensive than he had hoped. This was last night when I went to visit James, at around 7:30. What happened was that Dr. Gardiner told me this on the telephone as I was about to leave for the hospital. When I said I was coming he said he would elaborate in person. At the hospital I went to see James first. James told me "They didn't take my lung out." I was hurt and shocked that James had to know this in his weakened condition, for he had been opened up ... the whole surgical operation had been done, except for the removal of the lung.

Dr. Gardiner took me to a small room where we sat down. He told me that it had taken a long time in the O.R. to find the extent of the cancer, partly because the top lobe of the right lung had collapsed over the main part of the tumour. He told me they found that the cancer had spread beyond the lung to the trachea and the superior vena cava, and said there was extensive lymph node involvement. He wrote these things down for me. I asked him what stage the cancer had reached. Before, with the idea that it was confined to one lung and could be removed, it had been considered to be at what is termed stage I. Now Dr. Gardiner says the cancer is known to be at stage III B. I asked him if there was any such thing as a prognosis at this point, and he said he doesn't think Jim will live much more than a year. The big book Nancy sent confirms this. It gives the five-year survival rate for people with stage III B as less than five per cent.

Today James does not seem to be progressing well at all. He is very jaundiced, because of the liver's reaction to the extensive blood transfusions he has had during and since the surgery. He has a fever, and tonight he told me he needs oxygen almost continuously. He said, "I'm traumatized," and he repeated this; traumatized emotionally as well as physically, by the surgery and its futility.

July 17, 1992

Yesterday was a beautiful day studded in a long succession of rainy days. At a bus stop on the way to the hospital I saw a rhododendron tree in bloom in Bannerman Park, surrounded by beds of pansies, marigolds and stocks. The formality of the garden, the misty green trees, and a pecking starling and black dog sniffing, were miraculously beautiful in the face of what is happening. I realize that God is giving me a greater capacity to appreciate beauty, and it is a gift, the capacity, that he is giving me because I need it. Daisies, clover and a waterfall at the river on a walk with Esther this week gave me the same pleasure. I only pray now that God will give James something to gladden his heart too, and ease his pain and disappointment.

July 30, 1992

James is a lot better. The jaundice is gone, and he can do things for himself. Yesterday I bought a juicing machine and made carrot juice for him. I have read enough to convince me that more can be done to fight cancer than surgery and radiation. Nutrition, spirituality and the emotions have their part to play, too.

But we're having trouble with the emotional part. Our relationship has changed because for the past month I have been James' nurse, and because he may be dying. As his nurse, the role I've been given automatically is one of lifting him, cleaning his incision — which had become infected — making his bed, attending his toilet — all the things I used to do when I worked one time looking after old people. Doing that and caring for three-year-old Esther too, and dealing with the endless stream of visitors, all of whom require tea or coffee and some food and bright conversation ... Well, James wonders why I go to bed at 10:30, leaving him alone.

It's true that I have a lot of new feelings. Things are not the same as they were before he was diagnosed with cancer. Before we can have a spontaneous kiss or hug each other out of joy, delight or the happiness of little things in life, we have to step over the abyss of death. This is how I feel, anyway. Maybe it will change.

There is also this thought: if he really is going to die in a year, it is going to be very hard to live as if we weren't just waiting for death. The way we are used to feeling about our life has to change if it isn't going to be horrible. The way we are used to feeling — the way everybody feels — is that we assume we are building our life, our family, our relationships. I didn't realize until now how strong that feeling is ... and if the future is taken away from us, the whole point of the present is called into question. I have long heard that it is important to live in the present. I didn't know how very much my hopes were pinned on the future.

Most of the reason they are pinned on the future, I realize now, has to do with how dissatisfied I am about the present. I have been dissatisfied like this for some time — even before James' diagnosis. Now that I am writing this, my thoughts are sorting themselves out pretty fast. I would like to examine this, and then maybe — do something about it.

Both James and I have been having vivid dreams. Last night I dreamed there was a swan in the kitchen. I was busy, and I shooed it out the back door, where it stayed, pressing itself outside the kitchen window, pecking at the seam of the sill with its beak.

Now I feel that for me, as for others — because I have read it — a swan is the symbol of spiritual fulfilment. Graceful, mysterious, tall and beautiful, a swan can crown a pool with exquisite beauty. But this swan was out of the water; it was moving slowly and awkwardly across my kitchen floor, and its bottom feathers were dirty. Moreover I was much too busy to welcome this swan. I was answering a phone call, and someone was at the front door — a usual scenario these days. I told Jim of the dream at breakfast, just mentioning the swan's appearance and my herding it out the door, and he immediately said, "I would have kept it." That got me thinking about what the dream signified. I don't normally interpret dreams, but the meaning of this one seems pretty clear and simple.

A swan — symbol of spiritual fulfilment, and a creature I normally find beautiful — tried to come into my house. I noticed it was dingy and out of its element. I was too busy for it. I shooed it out. There is a certain person I need to become. I am not becoming her. I need to see the swan return to its magical pool and become fulfilled myself. The way is not clear yet, but it will become so.

September 27, 1992

Jim has tired easily and has been coughing ever since the last one or two radiation treatments. He is completely drained after any exertion and often has fits of a dry, hacking, itching cough. He came home today after visiting his family in Conception Harbour overnight, and I was struck by the fact that he looked unwell. The one-hour drive had drained him and he had to lie down immediately. He looked haggard and thin and drawn. I felt sad. He revived a little after he had a rest and I made him some food. I asked him if he thinks the fatigue and coughing are a result of the radiation or the cancer, and he said maybe it's both. Fatigue and coughing were symptoms he had before the operation or radiation.

Today was a perfect September day. Earlier, when Jim was still away, Michael and Gaile came to take Esther for awhile, but their itinerary was so inviting I went with them. We went walking in the hills above Quidi Vidi and found a table-shaped rock where we sat and had a picnic. The seams of the rock had partridgeberries sewn all down them, and in front of us, down below, the little inlet sparkled and glowed a deep green, while gulls wheeled and cried in the chamber of the rock inlet. The air was warm and scented. Esther and I took our shoes off and felt the warm rock, with its lichen.

Down below all around the water were people walking with babies, big-eared dogs, friends, each other. The whole town was celebrating a late September Sunday where the light struck trees' branches in a gold blaze and filtered through their leaves in a green haze. On a telephone wire six little birds sat up bright, watching. People who had fancy, old-fashioned cars paraded them with the tops down. It seemed not a leaf anywhere dared to turn yellow; all was green, summer held in suspension. I came home, and Michael and Gaile took Esther with them.

I read on the verandah for awhile, appreciating the trees draping the garden. Then I got out my new watercolours and did an ink and wash sketch of some fungus — which Esther with stunning accuracy says is like the dried apricots she likes to eat — growing out of the rotten old chopping block near the wood horse. Then I decided to walk to the end of the driveway to look at the lovely light that was gilding the trees and the western side of the street. At the bottom of the driveway I found the street irresistible, and so with the next street, until I was down by the river, walking and raising my arms to the lovely sun, the day, Sunday, in the straw hat Gaile had given me, a fringed goldy-brown scarf tied around the hat, and my new sunset-coloured dress. No wonder Jim looked unwell when he came back, compared to the gold light singing in my veins.

September 29, 1992

Jim is very sick today; fever, chills, weakness and fatigue, and pain in his lower back and head. He took some of the morphine elixir left over from his surgery. His cough is still bad, as it has been ever since the radiation stopped. He is lying on the couch under a sleeping bag all the time, and his eyes look sunken and his expression downhearted. At supper today he said, "I'm dying — my body is breaking down." I wonder how much of this is a reflection of other people's reactions to him — he says people treat him as doomed.

D with her husband L and son J came and took me and Esther partridgeberry picking. We went to the meadow we visited earlier this summer, and the partridgeberries were wine-ripe, glowing like jewels amid the caribou moss and around the junipers. The barrens beyond the meadows were rolling and fragrant under a blue sky. D and L brought their Coleman stove and we had a cup of tea on the berry grounds. Across the rolling hills we could see St. John's spread out, and two pockets of limitless ocean.

Then D and L took us to the other side of town to a trail in the woods, where we gathered chanterelles. It was the first time anyone had shown me how to identify these wild mushrooms, and to have been shown this is one of the highlights of my life. To me it is a very, very special thing to gather chanterelles. Their name alone describes their loveliness, delicateness and rarity. With their apricot-coloured stems flaring upwards in the peat floors of coniferous woods, they are, I told Esther, like fairy skirts dancing. I will sauté them

13

tomorrow in a little butter and share them with Michael and Gaile, as well as with my little family.

October 5, 1992

I'm at the Heritage Bakery Cafe. Jim is at home lying on the couch. Esther is at day care. I put her in all day today. I needed a break after the weekend. No day care on weekends. I realize, sitting here after eating a bowl of chili and bread and a muffin I didn't have to make myself or wash dishes after, that yesterday and today when I got out of the house and sat down somewhere, I was shaking. Yesterday I put it down to the nervousness of being a new driver — I'm driving to little sanctuaries now — but today I don't think it's just that. I've been out of the car forty-five minutes now, and I'm still shaky. This morning I felt impatient with Jim and tried not to show it, but he felt it. He just kept asking me to do little things — get him an apple, turn on the heat, sew buttons on his shirt à all reasonable things that I should do for him, but it seemed I couldn't get to sit down for a second, and after getting Esther ready and taking her to day care I just wanted everyone's claims on me to stop.

I managed to refrain from saying something very unkind to him. I said a wretched little prayer in the bathroom then went out and smiled at him. He smiled back. Everything's all right but it's perhaps more of a strain than I realize if I'm shaking when I get away. Later this morning as I was sewing buttons on my coat — that's when he quite reasonably asked if I'd do the ones on his shirt — he began to cry. He sobbed, lying there on the couch under the green quilt I got out of payment from a poetry reading and a brown scratchy woolen monk's blanket, and when I asked him to talk to me about it, he said, "It's Esther. I'm going to die and leave Esther."

"Little Esther," I said cruelly. He sobbed more.

"Her daddy." I was relentless.

"Yes. And she's too young."

I felt unsympathetic, although I stroked and comforted him.

"Maybe you won't die," I said. "Have you thought of that?"

"Yes."

"Do you think you're going to?"

"Yes."

I felt that if he died I wouldn't marry another man. I would get strong, and with Esther do the best I could to have a good, strong life in a cabin somewhere. I'd keep my friends, and I might get lovers, but I wouldn't marry anyone else. Either men are too dependent or they are bossy and manipulative. Today I just look at them and they fit right into one class or another. Either you end up having to look after them, or you wind up realizing they neither need nor love you.

Of course this is one of those momentary statements that life doesn't permit to survive. Poor Jim. Sometimes I think he'd be better off with his mother. She'd sew his buttons on, fuss over him, make him meals that he liked, love him more than I do. She wouldn't have other things on her agenda; selfish things, young woman things, wild river walks, sketchbooks and diaries. She wouldn't hurt him by having her own hidden, inner life.

October 6, 1992

Well, I'm at the Heritage Cafe again — for breakfast. Things are okay at home, but we are having some tense moments. Yesterday Jim said I never wanted to spend time at home. I said I just needed to get out and be alone sometimes, when Esther is in day care. It makes me feel good to sit over a coffee and write or read. At home it is too depressing if I have to stay there all the time. Jim does feel a little better this morning. I told him let's try not to let circumstances make our relationship deteriorate. I explained that I need time to recover, and that if I am not always solicitous to him it's because I find all this hard too. Actually I'm quite horrible. I just feel such a need to escape, especially now all of a sudden I have my driver's licence.

I love driving the car. Yesterday I took her to get a rim sealed and marvelled at how quickly the mechanic does heavy work, all his machines able to perform big tasks. He sprinkled water around the rim and found the leak and found one on the valve, too. He replaced the valve for nothing, and the whole job, which included lifting the car, locating the problem, removing the tire, sanding the rim and daubing rim and tire with sealant, replacing the valve, replacing the tire, replacing the wheel and lowering the car — cost me $5.99. I never saw anybody do that much work for $5.99 before. As he worked I thought of my brother, in Florida, doing the same

thing, with black hands, overalls and a mind full of dreams —
lifting a sunken sailing boat in the Bahamas, making enough
money to own his own garage in the Codroy Valley; never
saving any money, always getting into debt, trouble. Handsome to women and warmhearted, dangerous. I nearly cried
in the garage.

Driving a car. I love the car's privacy. You open the door
and get in, like a woman in a movie. You are in your own little
cubicle. The cubicle can move through the city, through the
country. Yesterday after my downtown errands I sat in the
car beside the parking meter and read a story in Gabrielle
Roy's *The Fragile Lights of Earth*. The car is a sanctuary, a
chariot of freedom, an escape vehicle. When I put the key in
the ignition and press the pedals, adjust the shift — all these
things are hard, mechanical, contrasted with my human and
female softness, yet they do what I say. No wonder men are
mad about cars. A car seals you off from the world, yet
through the world you spin, protected, enclosed. Not vulnerable like a walker, the cold wind blowing up your fingernails,
hurting the tender flesh inside your ears, torturing your face
and hair. A car makes you feel powerful. Of course, one
wrong move and you will see what a dangerous illusion this
is.

November 20, 1992

I'm at Woolworth's coffee shop now, where Santas, Snoopies
and presents are painted on the windows beyond which the
year's third snowfall is lightly floating across the big down-

town post office. A frowning woman with a short grey perm is drinking a huge soft drink in a paper cup, and her grandson takes it from her — it is his — and sucks so long and hard on the straw that his jawbone shakes.

Gradually Jim has come to the point where he goes outside only to do his weekly column or have a rare outing. The last outing was to go to Holyrood, where Gerry is making a clay sculpture of his head and shoulders. He hasn't been out since, except to do the column, and today if he has strength enough he wants to go out and buy a new pair of winter boots. I couldn't say, "What do you need boots for?"

I saw a mother, father and child walk past the decorated window in the snow of Water Street and felt a pang — will James, Esther and I ever walk like that again? Such a simple thing — as P says, people don't know what precious things they have.

Tuesday, January 12, 1993

Something glorious has begun to happen. The blockage that has prevented me and James, individually and together, from living the abundant life that Jesus promises, has begun to lift. Through the dark cloud shines a sun so bright, so warm, that it can heal anything. "Behold! The sun of righteousness will appear, with Healing in his wings!"

It is the dream of my heart that healing will occur, and God, the real god, the all-compassionate and all-creative, all-beautiful and loving one, god of tears and stars and oranges, will flow into people's hearts, and warm frozen places, healing wastelands of the human heart.

Healing wastelands of the human heart. D lent us some books. James is interested now in the inspirational videos, books and tapes he was too worn out to accept following the operation.

One of the books (by Lawrence LeShan) says what my swan dream said about healing. I know it is true for me as well, not just for anyone with cancer. He says cancer patients were all stifled at their hearts. For the first time James and I have been talking together about how love can flow in each of our lives, and in our lives together. I feel it has begun now.

The doll house I made for Esther, my painting classes, and now my Monday night meditation group, are all part of my new allowing of the heart to be free.

The doll's house I made for Esther is humble and lovely. All kinds of special dolls live there now. An orange-haired doll; a straw boy on a straw horse who plays near the little evergreen tree; a pink glass elephant; a little wooden cow; a porcelain deer — and an orange wooden boy who lies on a building block bed in the attic. In the night we turn the house front-on and Jim shines a small light inside so that the windows are lit up. It is alive and magical.

Jim has begun to let the love, light and magic flow for him, too. He is going to pay the small tuition debt he has owed the university for nine years. He is going to begin to take English courses, and work towards the degree he never finished. He is going to work towards being able to teach at the university. He told me today that not finishing is something he has always regretted, and that he believes he too needs to become the person he had stopped becoming. He became animated and very excited at the new plan. He became interested and motivated. He is going to visit our dear friends S and D in Cape Breton for a week at the end of January by himself. This is another thing he is doing for the inner James. We must allow our inner beings — our true selves — expression if we are to know healing. The selves our creator made us for. So much of the evil in the world is just this — the killing of the human spirit, which was meant to be full, joyous, abundant and godly. A small bit of me wonders what I will have to sacrifice, to allow Jim to work towards his dream, but god in me knows that only through his true fulfilment of who he was meant to be, and mine of who I am, and Esther's of who she is, can we allow love and healing to flow.

Wednesday, February 3, 1993

Early February in Newfoundland is not the best setting for one to achieve high spirits. Everywhere little nuggets of blackened salt, ice and slush litter the roads, which you have to walk on because the sidewalks are huge piles of the salt-ice-slush hardened stuff. Esther likes crushing these nuggets with her boots. I do too. The city's outside workers have been on strike for weeks, and the roads are covered in snow that has been assaulted and turned to a grimy mash by the cars that must travel to work anyway. Jim has been at S and D's a

20

week. He comes back tomorrow. A dry-run for when he dies, we joked; I'd see what is was like without him around. Well I suppose I'd survive. Anyway he's not dead yet.

I've been indulging in escape thoughts — a trip to Arizona, or New Mexico. The ochre earth colours and big spaces, vast stretches of desert sky, Indians.

I am on the rim between being young and old. Not young any more, but I tell myself I am younger than I will ever be again. A trip to New Mexico now would not be the thing it was when I went ten years ago. I sense I should be leaving the exploration experience and building, creating, with what I have amassed. But I would love an adventure. I realize an adventure can take place within one, without an outward journey, and until I can make my next outward journey I will try to journey — and adventure — inwardly. I was invited to give two journal-writing workshops to young people. Now I have been asked to do another in March. I learned things through my preparatory research and through being with the young people, who were forthcoming and generous with themselves. I think I can do more of these workshops, but I would like to develop them into something truly adventurous, and fruitful.

Fruitful ... that is the word of today. Abundant life. Not just making the best of things. I want to start making things happen. I've been an experiencer, a recipient of life. I have made the most of many opportunities, but now I want to step into the world of opportunity itself, be in the world of hope, sunrise, sunset, miracle ... swim in that element, not just reach for it from dry land, catching a few dewdrops.

Here in the February landscape the outer dreariness does not seem to lift nearly often enough. But I have always felt that need not spoil one's inner life. A trip to Arizona might help — somewhere charged with the particles of energy, possibility. But foremost these particles must be nourished in my own being. How? What must I do? Align myself with the Creator, that is the first thing. Yesterday, after a week of flu, as I began to feel better I felt lonely — having been stuck inside, without Jim — though with lovely Esther, bless her poor little heart — and I remember breathing ... even only imagining ... a very quite prayer that Creator might send me a flow of friends. N came ... we had a zucchini, tomato, onion, cheese and parsley omelette together, and a peaceful talk ... it was exactly what I needed. Then as I was nailing our bird feeder to a lilac branch, C dropped by ... he had just finished putting a bird feeder up at his new apartment. Then D came by, his head bandaged from his operation, his smile there, his knitting. A steady flow of friends ... from God. Thank you, Creator. So alignment with you is the first step in making something happen.

A woman is eating an orange at the next table. Alien to this civil servant coffee shop with its tiles and formica, flourescent lights and fabric ivy pots, it squirts and showers scent-spangles of freshness, citrus miracle, through the air.

A writing exercise with the non-dominant (left) hand as outlined in the book I found today: *The Well-Being Journal:*

Drawing on your inner power to heal yourself by Lucia Capacchione/ 1989.*

Right Hand: What is wrong with you, heart? What has been wrong with you all these years?

Left Hand: I am your heart. I am fine. There is nothing wrong with me at all, whatsoever. I am the best heart on earth. I am happiness, I am love, I am warmth, energy.

RH: Then why have you been in pain for years? I mean real, constricted pain?

LH: That's right, I've been constricted.

RH: How can I let you out free?

LH: See that? I mean feel that.

RH: Yes, you were holding the pen and a whole lot of pain just poured out, flooded out, disappeared, flowed out in a river, into the air, gone. Some is coming back now. Is that because I've got the pen? Was it just because you had the pen? I mean you weren't even saying anything. What will happen if ... I mean how can I learn to let the pain flow out?

LH: It feels good when I've got the pen, doesn't it? It feels like a big smile. This is my free and natural God-created state.

---

* This is a journal writing exercise in which the writer writes her own unsolved questions with her dominant hand — ususally the right —then uses the left, or non-dominant hand to write down the answers. Many people find that the left hand knows things the right hand doesn't. It often speaks for the forgotten heart, or inner self.

Energy rays. Lots of kisses and hugs. But this ... well, you do it.

RH: Okay, this is you — or what I think of as you — when you are constricted. Lots of fences and barbed wire. And I thought you were so intuitive and creative. (I thought I was.)

LH: You are. The barbed wire is not you ...

...It feels so good to do this. Here is a piece of freewriting by my heart:

> big slow dripping
> raindrop off a warm
> twig in spring
> feeds the furled
> leaf inside the
> sheath,
> makes it sticky
> fertile bud
> scented with
> divine
> fragrance
> of earth
> rainwater
> sap
> and sun
> I am your heart

February 4, 1993

RH: What are you feeling today, heart?

LH: I flow, like a divine stream, even as the sleet drives. Yes,

I can help you to love Jim. You know how, pretty good.
But I would not deny myself in the process. He needs to
love you too.

RH: I'm concerned that this is pretty silly. You know, ridiculous.

LH: Creator must be ridiculous too then. All those desert
sunsets just for the sake of beauty, loveliness.

Jesus — the Christ — remember where, in the faith-given
one, the Christ resides.

RH: In the heart. In my heart. So it's okay to listen to you?
Maybe if I ask Jesus — Yeshua — to speak to me through
my heart ... but which is me and which is Yeshua?

LH: He said I and the Father are one and you are in him and
he in you. You are the branch and he is the vine. Let the
holy spirit flow through you.

RH: I'm scared of giving up control.

LH: That is the battle. Not works, but faith. Trust. Resting in
the leaf-boat of your God.

RH: I'm afraid all this is not true.

LH: Keep connected. I am here. I am with you.

February 6, 1993

Today we drove to St. Michaels and visited Vicky and Mrs.
Tee. At Vicky's it was Jesse's first birthday. There were other
friends, and lots of kids. Vicky harnessed a wheeled sleigh to
Freida, her St. Bernard dog, and we took the kids for a sleigh
ride toward Bauline.

As we went along, the adults walked ahead and behind

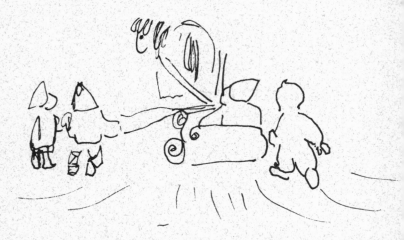

the bundle of children. The dog, sleigh and children were a
bundle of wonderfulness ... Esther and Miles held the reins
while first Ivor and then Kate rode. Then Esther had a ride.
The little collection of dog, sleigh, riding child and rein-hold-
ing children, self-sufficient and not in need of us, was a
trundling delight.

The Friday night party was another success. I went alone.
Jim rested after his Nova Scotia trip.

He came back in a beautiful dark wool greatcoat that
he'd found in a second-hand store for six dollars. Then we
went down to Chafe's men's store to get him a hat, and we got
a Russian hat, a great wild Russian hat of bear fur or some
wild animal ...in this magnificent hat and beautiful coat Jim
cuts quite a figure. He's very pleased with himself and it's
great to see him looking so good. He looks quite dramatic,
and he knows it.

Friday, February 12, 1993

I am not minding this February at all. The sun has come out many days in a row, and there is bright, soft, new, clean snow in a healthy thick coat everywhere. The trees are graceful in their spreading reaches and the roads are covered in a pale frost coat because the striking city workers have stopped mucking them up with salt and sand. To walk somewhere is to move briskly in dancing light, frost sparkles spiralling in the air, pure, fresh air washing one's breathing. Jim is like an Arctic explorer this morning in his Russian hat, fur-hooded parka and old green knapsack, dusty green corduroy trousers, as he heads off to class and the library.

Last night I dreamed he died. They took his body away somewhere before I had seen it. I travelled all over the hospital and the city, which had become unfamiliar, looking for the doctor, the room where Jim lay. I searched with Esther in my arms. We couldn't find him. I have never felt such a sense of loss as I did in that dream. No matter how much anybody — friends, family, hospital staff — cared or helped us, nobody loved us like Jim. Nobody understood us like Jim, and we didn't love or understand anyone like we loved him. I cried in the dream, and it was a deep, tragic wailing cry from the soul. It was one of those dreams whose feelings are true when you are awake, too. I awoke and snuggled into him. I never told him about the dream. He snuggled back.

"I had a good dream," he told me. He dreamed a man gave him a book. The man had had cancer but the cancer had

27

been overcome, the man cured. The book was about how this had happened.

"You can do it too," the man told Jim. Jim felt good about the dream. I was glad. Jim told me about another dream last week. He and his brother Gord were fishing. They caught a giant, dangerous eel, and killed it. I think they cut its head off. Later, when they went to go fishing again, all the water had dried up out of the lake. Gord had just quit smoking. I interpreted the dream to mean that Gord and Jim slew cancer together. The lake drying up meant the element in which the cancer lived had dried up, and the cancer could live no longer.

Here I want to document what I know about the physical things that may have contributed to Jim's cancer. He smoked cigarettes for years. When I first knew him he often smoked home rolled cigarettes of Drum tobacco without filters.

Sixteen years ago he worked for four months at the Canadian Gypsum plant in Calgary, making plastic pipes. He told me he mixed compounds together, the ingredients of the plastic. One of these ingredients created a lot of dust. Jim says he thinks it contained PCBs. Someone had drawn a skull and crossbones on the wall over these ingredients. Masks were provided to be worn by the workers but Jim never wore one. He broke out in boils when he worked there and was given time off because of them, without question. Jim says that may have been because the company knew the compounds were responsible for the boils. Jim has had boils before. He is prone to them. The stuff he mixed was yellowish crystals and black pellets, he said. The mixture would be put through a machine called an extruder, and lengths of plastic "mud" would come out into baths of cold water, where they would harden in the shape of the plastic pipes that were the company's product.

Jim's eating habits have always been what I would call pretty bad. He ate nitrite-laden bologna all his life. He has always drunk Coke. He likes fried food and lots of meat, and does not like carrots or squash or many of the other foods abundant in beta-carotene, although he does like turnip and cabbage as well as brussels sprouts. He eats white bread. Whole grains, beans, fresh vegetables and fruit are not in his diet very much at all. He loves apples and eats a lot of them. He is a fiend for coffee with sugar, and has drunk a lot of instant coffee for years. He is a fiend for sticky buns and peanut butter cookies — all kinds of cookies and baked goods.

I am not writing this down to blame Jim for his cancer. But I am bearing witness to some factors that I believe may be connected to it. He is eating good food with me now. Since he came back from Nova Scotia where S practices macrobiotics, we have begun again to eat many whole grains with simple vegetables, although I am providing occasional meat and am still buying sweet fruit. Yesterday I made peanut butter cookies with unpasteurized wildflower honey and whole wheat flour. It would be better if we could go without them but I feel they are better than cafeteria dutchies.

I have so much more energy on this grains and vegetables diet. Last night I went for a walk in the crystal starlight.

Usually by the time Esther gets put to bed I am too pooped to do anything. She goes to bed around 8 p.m. When I came back last night from my invigorating walk, Jim was watching the Bernie Siegel video "You Can Fight For Your Life," that we got from the cancer support group. I felt so good about that.

I'm glad I had the dream. I needed to know just how much I would miss him. He needs to know it. The dream will help me to show him, help me to show him love more.

I have been thinking about the journal writing workshop I have been asked to do with high school students. I've been thinking I should make it inspirational. So many Newfoundland kids get lost in a quagmire of TV sitcoms, processed food and dead-living so early that it's a tragedy. The whole dead core in our culture as a people is a tragedy. The death of confidence, imagination, ideas and health in our society is a tragedy, a terrible evil. I am thinking about how I can do a workshop that explores how to use journal writing as a way to fight death in life and become as alive — spiritually, mentally, physically — as it is possible for each one to be. That should be fun for both me and the kids. I can show how to use journal writing to identify and wash away the things that are wearing you down. How to use it to ask spiritual questions and find a path that leads to God. How to use it to listen to yourself, your true self, in a world where many voices say wrong, unhealthful things. Kids need to hear this. They need to hear they should seek God until they find him and her. That freedom, truth and joy are their birthright.

Wednesday, February 17, 1993

Today James felt some symptoms that, coupled with a recurrent pain in his right side, make him wonder if the cancer might have spread to his liver. He was tired this evening and went to bed at 9:30, just a few minutes ago. He never goes to bed early. I know that with cancer one never knows if a feeling is a cancer symptom or not. For some reason tonight I feel more alarm than usual about this sign. Is it a sign, or is it just nothing? On the desk in front of me is a beautiful, peaceful angel, a photograph taken by our friend David of a cemetery angel. Her hand is resting over her heart (James says angels are men. I say they're just angels but I like to call them she), and her face has an incredibly gentle look. The stone angel — an image of stillness and peace.

March 12, 1993

I decided in these journals I was going to at least try not to apologize for my feelings. What would be the point? A big part of cancer is the uncertainty and slowness with which it does its work, and I have feelings about that. When he dies … if he dies … uncertainty. Meanwhile I am supposed to remain concerned about him only, happy to remain loyally at his side whether he lives, dies, fluctuates, swindles, pines or thrives, all the while unconcerned about the eventual outcome, concerned not for myself, my sexual life, passions, youth, age, companionship — for it is a very certain kind of companionship I enjoy now; one in which Cancer comes to bed with us, sits in the apartment with us, laughs, hides coyly, doesn't come out with a statement of its intentions, expects me to ignore it, love it, console it, like being with it. Well, I don't like being with it, and I do feel that its slowness is a horrible thing, not a blessing. Today that is what I feel, and I make no apology about it.

Sunday, March 21, 1993

I need this journal for healing tonight. It's funny; I got used to telling Jim everything, and now that he is dying he has become part of what confronts me; part of the "other," and I can no longer confide in him completely. I'm trying to get a grip on myself and "face it."

"Face it" is what I learned today at my old-time haunt, Ladies' Lookout on Signal Hill. Ladies' Lookout is a stone seat in a cleft in the cliff face at the top of Signal Hill. I drove up to Signal Hill today and walked past the tourists to the lonely place. Today was a glorious day welcoming spring. The snow's crust surface had blue fire in it and flashing ruby crystals. In Ladies' Lookout I found some comfort in the cold cliff face. The rock had two streamlets of melting ice trickling from one crevice. Splotches of cheerful lichen adorned the stone seat, on which I sat looking out to sea. I gathered sticks, a dried flower star, soft yellow-brown grasses.

I regarded the stone face rising over me into the sky with comfort. The cold air, cold stone, cold me. I felt good. The stone was "facing it," and I must face it, too. The stone wasn't indulging in any illusions or delusions. I must be like that, too. The gifts of dry thistle and grasses, melting streamlets like tears down the rock, lonely bird calls; all were strong, and I must be strong. Some tears glistened down my face, too.

I gathered my mosses and thistles and grasses (the grasses were laid low, hugging the earth), and I pressed my lips to the cliff face. I was surprised. It was the best kiss I've had in years. Who would have thought the rock of a cliff so passionate.

Tonight I went to the Cathedral with a friend, and the service was about the link between passion and suffering. I could relate to that. Lent is accompanying me with its beautiful story of fasting and barrenness, passion and suffering, cold rock and flesh pressing against each other in an embrace of love and agony.

Wednesday, March 24, 1993

Last night I dreamed he died. He was being cremated. To do this he stood in a large room in a funeral parlour and followed

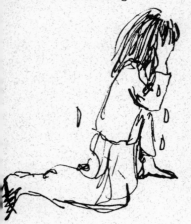

the instructions of a man in front of the room. (He could still follow the instructions even though he was dead.) At the right moment he turned into a neat little pile of ashes. He was gone. I went outside and walked down the street. Then I woke up and he was still alive.

I feel I need a place to call my own, a place that is not sewn to Jim and cancer. Today I feel close to breaking down emotionally. The demands are impossible to fill, and there is no joy. Perhaps I will be able to look back on this and see it's the cancer that is causing these pressures. Now I just feel weary, worn and sick of it, and of course, I feel guilt.

Sunday, 28 March, 1993

The day after the last entry things between us became okay again. I guess more things affect us than we know. The weather, hormones, moods, "pressure systems." Spring has come, with shining rivulets of melting ice-water on the roads, the scent of trampled earth, vast warm skies with creamy clouds.

Thinking of buying the Holyrood house.

C, a dear man from the church we used to attend, died of cancer two weeks ago. We were told today. C was diagnosed with a brain tumour after Jim was diagnosed. Jim feels depressed about C's death. Jim has been "caught up" in the chest now for a few days, coughing and wheezing, not badly, but any amount is alarming.

Wednesday, April 7, 1993

Your House:

S, this morning the sun was blazing, and I knew I had to go to your house. The past few days have been hard for me. Pressures and responsibilities have overwhelmed me. I was in such bad shape I was nearly having accidents in the car,

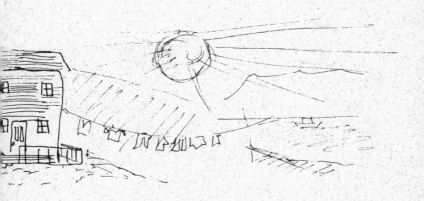

and I was shaking, and doing things like locking the keys in the car. I couldn't think. I felt things were demanded of me that were unrealistic and impossible. I felt life was just too hard. My heart was very, very sore. I had been crying a lot, and feeling very unstable, weak; near collapse. I knew that the morning sun beats down on your wooden verandah. I had only twenty free minutes before I had to resume my family and work responsibilities, which I felt I couldn't face. I drove to your house, parked the car, and walked up your wooden steps. I sat on a step and closed my eyes, turning my face to the warm sun. The sun has just started to feel warm after the winter.

One of the cats that find shelter in your house had plonked himself on the wooden railing above me. He too was letting the sun's warmth sink into his body. We were both the same, hugging the warmth, enjoying the feeling of sanctuary that surrounds your house as well as existing inside it. I felt so glad to be near you. The feeling of love and acceptance that surrounded me when I thought of you was healing, like the sun on the warm wood. Right now, I thought, this is the one place I can go to and be totally accepted, where I can be completely myself. Because myself is pretty weird right now. She goes to your verandah and sits there in the sun like a cat, her eyes closed (but tears are slipping out), praying for strength and getting it, from your house, the sun and warm wood, the beautiful washing dancing on the line up the road, the silence broken by the sounds of gulls and a few morning voices calling the dog and the children, the smell of the ocean, the beautiful fresh wind, just a breeze, with fresh coolness riding on the warmth. Here I don't have to do all the right things, I can just be me and be loved. I knew that this place of unconditional love and acceptance was reality and truth, and all places where these gifts are banished are unreality and falsehood, and this knowledge made me stronger as I sat and received it.

After I was finished praying for strength for myself I prayed for strength, love, healing for you, the cats, and all who might come here or be touched by you this day. I felt blessing all around me there, and left a small kiss on the banister as I left to go home. Such a house of love is a rare thing, and a light, and a comfort to all who pass by, seeking.

Tuesday, April 27, 1993

Here is one of the beautiful segments of the Song of Solomon that I can't bear —

The Shulamite

"My beloved is white and ruddy,
Chief among ten thousand.
His head is like the finest gold;
His locks are wavy,
And black as a raven.
His eyes are like doves
By the rivers of waters,
Washed with milk,
And fitly set.
His cheeks are like a bed of spices
Like banks of scented herbs.
His lips are like lilies
Dripping with liquid myrrh.
His hands are rods of gold
Set with beryl.
His body is carved ivory
Inlaid with sapphires.
His legs are pillars of marble
Set on bases of fine gold.
His countenance is like
Lebanon,
Excellent as the cedars.
His mouth is most sweet,
Yes, he is altogether lovely.
This is my beloved,
And this is my friend,
O daughters of Jerusalem!"

Friday, April 30, 1993

A few things have happened to return to me the gift of being able to love my husband. The terrain of the heart is so mysterious, it is impossible to say with certainty what the things are exactly, or even if it is these things and not some mysterious wave or current. However I do love James today, and prize and cherish him, and I am grateful and relieved to be able to do so ... to see him for his best, loveliest, most spiritual and poetic self. His soulful self, the one that I married. And of course to do that I have to become my soulful self, the one that married him.

First of all, Gerry gave James a portrait done as he sat in the class Gerry was instructing. The portrait is the nicest one, I think, that he has done of James. In it Jim's face, hair and expression are bathed in a soft light. Gerry has captured Jim's thoughtfulness, gentleness, his poetic and spiritual soul, and his feelings as he faces death: acceptance of it and sorrow about his youth, dying young and leaving a wife and Esther.

I have come into the other room to look at the portrait as I write about it. The head is filled with thoughts, and they have the strength and sadness I just mentioned. But there is also the feeling that Jim is not alone. The light that is coming, just small, but soft and strong, from the side he faces ... and the vulnerable, accepting aloneness of his face, and the beautiful colours — dark blue-black and warm, deep purple — of his clothing ... this is the beautiful Jim, the one whom God is with. One cannot doubt, in looking at the painting, that his God is with him. All the human problems, the petty things, fall away when faced with the ultimate eternal spirituality of the person. I can see that Gerry has put himself in the painting, too, because he also has, as Jim has sometimes, this beautiful, strong, pure quality about him — this clarity and transparent truthfulness, as a clear pond lets you see into its beauty — its fish, rocks, green underwater life. Gerry knows, best of all people perhaps, how to understand or at least see this special duality Jim has — on the one hand this clear, striking quality, and on the other hand the muddied waters, the clouded view, the life clouded with cares that lead to sin, as the Bible calls our manifest weaknesses. But in this painting is the lovely quality of forgiveness — this is James with his forgiven soul, as Jesus sees him, as Jesus, saying "Judge Not," would have all of us see each other.

Then Beth called this morning. She is one of the world's fairest natural objects, like a star, or a beautiful stone, a gem. She spoke about how I will speak to Jim after he dies, when I look up at the stars, and he will not seem far from me.

And there is the weather: soft, misty, rainy; forgiving and healing, mysterious and comforting in its dimness, no glare.

Then there are the tidal pulls, the moon's influence on my woman tides; as they change so do my inner oceanic waves ... This whole experience between James and myself has taught me how influential these pulls beyond my will, my conscious control, are upon me. I humble myself before this knowledge, love it and forgive myself.

Later:

I don't believe a woman has ever discouraged me from anything. Whereas I was just at a friend's house and I noticed her man discouraged her about several things. Then she fell asleep (discouraged altogether?) whereupon he began to try and discourage me. He found three things to discourage me about, and then he left.

It took some time to reassure myself. Then I came home and my man began to discourage me about a whole different set of things. I came in here (the bedroom) with the door locked, and began to think of the women I know who have men, and I realized the men keep discouraging them. Then I thought about how my women friends are with me. They encourage me.

So I went out and told Jim I've decided not to let anybody discourage me again. He gave a derisive grunt. So I've come in here with the door locked to record this announcement, this observation.

The scheme is found out now. When I think of it I'm sickened at the way men try to discourage women from doing all kinds of brave, interesting, courageous things. Oh I hate my husband tonight. He said I never sew his buttons on so I'm not a real woman-wife. He tries that one every now and then, and it always takes me by complete surprise. The injustice he feels! The seriousness of it to him! Oh I could take his buttons and stuff him with them.

May 03, 1993

Tonight for the script project I went to the home of a young Bengali woman who performed a sacred classical Indian dance for me, and played and sang a song by Rabindranath Tagore, playing on the Indian instrument the harmonium, in the temple in her home. One of the lines from one of the songs was, ruin my sin, destroy it, take it from me. She is not a Hindu but follows one of the gurus who claim to be manifestations of God and preach love and unity of all religions. Her mother made me coffee and malpua, a sweet cake with cardamom. Again I found myself in a place with a person totally unusual to me yet beautiful. And always the reality of Jim's cancer, his closeness to death, underlies these things; another unusual and off-centre thing; it's as if everything has thrown off the pretense of being balanced; cast off the garment of predictability to reveal something — a life — filled with amazing, unknown elements. More now I lose the feeling of being able to control my life, the illusion that I know the stuff of which it is made, the course it should take, the rightness of things. Ruin my sin, she said the dance was saying, and the phrase was so beautiful, and so was the dance.

Jim phoned as I was writing this — in the warm breeze on the verandah at our soon-to-be-left 16 Argyle, surrounded by lilac and maple trees about to bud — and we had a warm, companionable conversation. It feels so good to be able to enjoy him again, to be coming free. The birds sing. Summer is coming. What is going to happen? Only god knows.

Even god experiences surprise.

Tuesday, May 11, 1993

I'm at Tim Hortons. It's night time. Some women, blessed and magical because they are in their sixties, have sat at this table. I know this is an illusion born of ignorance but I feel such a relief in their presence; everything is so much of a burden for women my own age, and for those in their forties and fifties too. By the time these women have reached their sixties, they are wearing dresses made of fabric covered in roses. Their voices are no longer soft and yielding — but are starting to sound papery. When there is a group of them as there is here, tonight, they appear, each one, to have clear air around them, not a cloud of domestic worries, the heaviness that surrounds middle-aged women. I picture them having interests that require concentration, a rolling up of sleeves, a tying back of hair with long scarves.

Tonight I prepare to read portions of this journal — to record them — for a CBC radio's Morningside. Morningside asked me, through Marie, to prepare a final paragraph — "about moving to the country, about how Jim has exceeded all the doctors' best expectations" etc. "You want a happy ending," I laughed on the phone. "No," she told me, "be true to yourself." So as far as I can be, I will. I can't write a happy ending of course, but I was going to record something that happened last night between me and James.

I was feeling so miserable — heavy hearted. War-torn over the cancer, depressed and overwhelmed at the amount of work — and moving house — that I face. Mostly though I was feeling tormented in my heart over the fact that here were James and I in the same room — together in life — and I didn't love him. Somehow we began to talk about this. I told him I didn't love very many people at all. He asked me if I loved Esther and I said no. I said she never does what I ask — she makes demands — she is one big demand. I don't feel love in my heart. On one hand a person who doesn't feel love for her terminally ill husband or her four-year-old child may seem to be a horrible person. But from her point of view — my point of view — it's torture not to feel love. It hurts to be unable to love. James said, "You do love Esther," — and he told me about the times he's seen me hug her, kiss her, love her pudgy cheeks. I do love her big pudgy hands, her pudgy feet. I suppose I love bits of her and bits of him. But everyone wants me to write about "the marvellous gift of hope," and I don't want to. I'm sick of telling people how well Jim is doing, sick of describing the state of his health.

Anyway, back to last night. Instead of getting hurt at my lack of love, Jim sympathized. He was helpful. And he said something that revolutionized the way I've been looking at the cancer, at our marriage. He said that because of the cancer we are not the same couple we were before it happened; we are really a different couple. And he's right.

And it's because I've been looking at us as the same couple — injured and war-torn — that I've felt so miserable. Looking at us as the old us — with cancer — is not the same as looking at us as a whole new couple. If I look at us as a new couple altogether, I see new possibilities. No longer is the future a failed version of our hopes. The future does not begin with the old couple, the past. It begins with us the way we have become. Our old hopes might be dead. It's time to see that they are dead, and to bury them. To start from now, instead, presents us with a whole new set of possibilities. I merely begin to understand this now as I write.

Intuitively I feel our moving to the country fits in with this. Our old hopes, our old dreams, our old selves, each and together; buried. But Jim is still here, and I am still here, and Esther is just starting out, but even she faces this change. We are still here, and we have survived everything that has happened to us. If we continue with the tattered forms of our old selves, we will be pathetic and wounded and eternally sad. I don't understand this fully yet, but perhaps Jim is right, and we have changed, each of us and together, into someone, something, else. Somehow I feel this insight equips us for our new future, our different future, the one we never thought we would have.

Monday, May 24, 1993

New leaves have just begun to greenly feather branches all over St. John's. As I passed Rawlin's Cross I came by the laburnum tree that I have noticed every year since I came to town after living in St. Michael's. I link the tree with James Joyce's poem "Alone" in Pomes Penyeach:

The moon's grey golden meshes make
all night a veil:
The shore-lamps on the sleeping lake
laburnum tendrils trail.
A sly reed whispers to the night
a name — her name;
and all my soul is a delight,
a swoon of shame.

When I passed the laburnum this morning it came to me
how much I have experienced since I first saw it — how old I
have grown while it remains as graceful, as lovely, as tanta-
lizing as it did when I felt youthful and relatively carefree. I
know time gives us the illusion that things were more beautiful in the past than they really were, but I still felt this regret,
this feeling that I was weighted down with the cares of the
world while the laburnum tree was the same as before.

After the laburnum tree comes a segment of LeMarchant
Road that has the same kind of enchantment for me in my life.
At this section of the road one can look beyond a wire fence
and see the city descending in stages or steps to the water,
then the ships and water, and lights on the water ... and the
whole scene is just like one of those books whose scenes raise
themselves three-dimensionally when you open them up,
very magical. This magical part of the city came right after the
romantic laburnum tree, and between these two I saw a
young tree feathering its new pale green spring leaves in
front of an old blue evergreen in a garden — it made me
breathless, the way it shared its new green leaves, so soft, like

big soft snowflakes — and it was as if they could melt, they were so soft and new.

As I came to the special scene of the descending city, thinking of the laburnum and of the breathtaking, blossoming tree, two bitter tears came to my eyes. To think how the city was remaining the way it was when I was young and carefree and romantic, and now I was so worn, and yet the city was breaking forth in another new spring. I felt how much more like this must old people feel; an old woman, an old man; grown truly old in a city where they were young once. I am only thirty-three, came the thought; maybe when this is all over you can be young again, you can have another spring in which you are young and carefree, and even romantic. But I felt old and worn all the same, and the two little tears stung and dried up; they didn't overflow like young, romantic tears do.

Thursday, July 1, 1993

Tomorrow will be a year to the day since James was admitted to the hospital. I write this as a lace curtain sweeps past the window in the loft bedroom at our new home in Holyrood, the little black house we have bought, the place where we came last summer and stayed two nights to see what it felt like. The window is open: beyond I can hear the stream that lulls us to sleep. Downstairs the woodstove has a birch fire in it despite the date. Here there is still cool mist on the hills, and rain, coolness. The fire feels good. Jim feels fine. He has a

46

small cough. He is fat and cheerful. I am grateful to God for giving us this house.

The wild flower book I mentioned at the start of this journal — which I said I wished this journal could be — perhaps its time is coming. I started a new journal soon after we moved here. I am noting flowering plants and nature notes in it. So far I have seen pink lady slipper orchids, ospreys and their nest, and Clintonia lilies and wild lily-of-the-valley. All these plants have medicinal uses according to my Peterson guide. The wildflower society is having a field trip near here in July, and I plan to go. I'm researching wild flower entries for volume five of the Newfoundland Encyclopedia. Flowers and medicines for the heart, my ravished heart; my heart is like the centre of a wild rose — its petals have been torn off by the cruel winds. But God is at my centre; no, faith is at my centre; faith in the God who blows the winds, who creates me, who knows why I love whom I love, who knows by heart the fragrance of roses and the mutilating thorns.

July 6, 1993

I'm in Toronto for the first time, for CBC workshop. The workshop is great but they put us up in the Holiday Inn and today I left there and moved my stuff to the Marigold Travellers' Hostel on Dundas St. West. It's a dive but there's an intelligent guy downstairs operating it with Shirley whose wrists are covered in medical bracelets, her hands full of brown plastic pills jars — she kissed and hugged me. The other inhabitants are Jose from Mexico and someone from France. Mattresses on the floor and rickety bunks, but you can hear the streetcars and the rain through the open window. The pink corners of "my" room are slanted and kittycornered, and beyond a tattooed woman reading there is an open door leading to a thunderstorm-drenched wooden balcony that the proprietor, intelligent amid the squalor, said I could use. (I'd been wondering if I could use it since the tattooed woman's reading chair was propped in the doorway — with her in it. I think her name is Joanne).

I'm in the Greek bar on the corner drinking draft beer, about to order deep fried calamari, a Caesar salad and garlic bread. To get to the Marigold I took the Dundas St. West streetcar from Spadina just as the thunderstorm hit after days of sultriness. The streetcar was tortuously beautiful, creaking and settling its way along the necklace of lit-up Portuguese bakeries, shops and balconied homes with fox-gloves and tomato plants in vegetable-box front yards ... women in cotton housedresses mopping their balconies after the rain.

I took myself toward High Park after I checked in, looking for something to eat, and passed Halal's goat general grocery where yellow boards with red painted words proclaimed 2 Baby Goats —$99.00, 2 Medium Goats $128.00, and a dingy canvas sign, sagging from wetness, further encouraged me to buy the same two baby or medium goats and get one free.

I saw a little second-hand shop and bought a beautiful old amethyst set in a golden heart with twining leaves for

$8.00. The man in there was sweet. After I had bought it he turned it around in his hand and said it's a very old piece and it might be a real amethyst because the back isn't silvered, which they do with fake ones. Amethyst is my birth-stone. Amethyst is magic to me. I can't tell the difference between amethyst now and amethyst in my childhood. When I was in Naples I bought a little amethyst elephant and gave it away. The little heart reminds me of Naples, of courage in a strange land, of adventure, of the thrilling loveliness of San Francisco, Naples, streetcars in Portuguese neighbourhoods in Toronto.

I had to get out of the $90.00 per night Holiday Inn on King Street — the most evil place I have ever been in — the most evil, evil, evil place. My squid are here. Lovely calamari, of Picasso, of Bracque, of Greece, of Italy, of Newfoundland. The food is passionate. That place — the Holiday Inn — for a start, they treat you like shit. I don't know what people like about it. It's cold, lifeless, featureless; dead and evil; enough to chill your bones and blood. Enough to kill you. The elevators, the pale brown carpets, the cold city lights out the window, the air conditioning, the stupid little coffee machine and hair dryer and little bottles of shampoo and packets of soap — the mirrors, the beds big enough for four people, the stupid newspaper they put on the desk, the incredibly stupid room service that gives you three muffins when you ask for one, and comes in and throws away the one you were saving for breakfast. All the stupid little adolescent kids with fish on their shirts and gel in their hair; the stupid front desk with its obsequious wardens of idiot decorum. I'm ecstatic I'm out of there and in here with the calamari and beer, my old gold amethyst heart leafwoven, and the couple who are embracing across the room; she is wide-hipped, with shaggy bleached hair; he is brown with a black beard and black strap shirt, his arms around her with love. Streetcars go by, here with the calamari, where things are magical and full of life.

Wednesday, July 21, 1993

Jim has a cold. He says he can feel himself "slowly dying — if this is how sick I get when I have a cold."

Yesterday I howled in the car on the drive from business meetings in town to Holyrood. I cried, howled and screamed. I cried like Esther cries, tears and rage and tragedy. I prayed in a way I've never prayed; all pretensions at holiness gone. I swore at God, cursed and screamed, told him and her everything I was mad at. I was a person who broke promises; a bad person, awful — an absolute wreck. I've been joking that when we got married "Charlie Chaplain" should just have said for worse, for poorer, in sickness — and not bothered with the rest.

I told God I couldn't bear things for one more second. I burst with frustration, and when I got home a miracle happened. Esther was there in a lime coloured dress I've never seen before — just vibrant, her hair with the bangs grown out and swept to one side; Jim was in the pre-Raphaelite shirt and vest I'd got him in Toronto, and he looked beautiful. They shimmered, they both did. I was coming home to the best family anyone could have.

I can feel sad now not because of Jim and his cancer, but for all the things that could have been between us in the future — our life. Things that won't be. I haven't felt that for a long time, and it feels good. I felt it at the beginning of this whole cancer journey, but then pressures got in the way.

I'm waiting in the King's Bridge Hotel for a 9 a.m. appointment with N, a counsellor with the Anglican family life office. This hotel is old and friendly. I saw some town things on the drive in here — an old woman putting her garbage out; a little brother and big sister playing on a shady verandah with a stick.

I called N in January. She's free so that's why it's not until now that I can see her. But now is a good time. I believe in seeing a counsellor if that's what you want; someone impartial who is paid to do it, who you won't be burdening, who you can tell things you might not feel like telling the various people close to you.

I visited the Centre, the mental health activities centre that T and the residents at H talk so much about. The place is park-like with a greenhouse and friendly staff — they are short-staffed. I offered to do something. S there said please do. He said I could do my own workshops or dance with the guys at dances or help serve food at the barbecues. Maybe I'll just go there and listen. Yesterday before I cried, I couldn't catch my breath. I can breathe now.

August 16, 1993

We had some strawberry, trout and canoe days. Esther and I dived and splashed in the green water of Butterpot Pond. My mother and father visited and fixed the pump and climbed Butterpot Mountain with me. I sat on a blanket with Nina and my mother and watched gold and blue meteors trail smoky plumes across the sky. In the necklace of occasional dreams came one where I was told I had cancer. I then knew how it felt. For me it felt as if my life was spoiled, and there was some shame and disgrace connected to it. Spoiled, my life that had held such promise and newness. All youth was gone, and a heavy stone sat in my heart.

Boy on the bus: Nanny, tell me what you used to look like
   when you were one year old.
Nanny: I don't know. It's a long time since I was one year old.
Boy: Tell me!

In my little Ruskin book I read this, this morning:

> *The White-Thorn Blossom*
> *(Fors Clavigera, Vol. 1, Letter 5)*
>
> For lo, the winter is past,
> The rain is over and gone,
> The flowers appear on the earth,
> The time of the singing of birds is come,
> Arise, oh my fair one, my dove
> And come.

The day after I had the dream, I felt a kind of awful love for Jim; felt how disappointed he must feel; this is his one and only life, and he has been told it is lost.

I felt his loss, and I was able to forget myself. But it was just for a day. I am not able to be saintly about this.

Jim is dying. And I have the power to make his dying days happy. But I don't have the power at all. I am powerless. I fall in love with other men. I am ignoring it. The cancer. Trying to cut it — and Jim out of my life. Unsuccessfully. And making a mess.

Wednesday, September 15, 1993, 10:05 a.m.

Esther is playing with bread dough. She is making characters from Circle Park: Matty, Danny, Sylvia and herself ... the bedtime story I tell her (a long serial — the other one is Rat Belfry, for contrast and fun). Bread is rising. We have just made muffins with fresh blueberries. Yesterday some script work came in. It will be a lot of work over the next few weeks. Esther will have to go to day care. I came home yesterday and was feeling sad at having her go. When I came in she was lying on her belly on the kitchen floor, saying, "I've got no one to play with and I'm cranky." Jim is in bed. He feels nauseous. He says he felt so last night too.

Today I feel such love for our little house and family in the woods, baking bread inside, the soft air outside hanging blue in the trees. Still and quiet. Yesterday when I left Esther was still asleep, her rosebud pudgy face in the crook of Jim's

("Fuzza dada's") neck. I know I am going to feel such remorse after he is dead — if he dies — I still have to say that; still feel maybe he isn't going to. One of my books on journals suggests one might see if one tends to write in crisis or in peace. I have written a lot in crisis, and maybe there's too much about the bad parts of our relationship. There are good parts too. Today is such a soft, homemade day, and I feel so strongly the preciousness of such a time, and I keenly feel my love and appreciation for Esther and Jim, our pussy cat, woodstove, sack of whole-wheat flour, sound roof, and the blue air through the trees.

I've long wanted to record that special look Esther has sometimes, and she had it when I looked at her sleeping with Fuzza Dada early yesterday morning. It's a mature look. Her cheeks slope down from the little inlets under her eyes in a droopy, pendulous slope. Her little head is held high on her sweet neck, high and grave, very grave for a little four-year-old. I mentioned it to Michael yesterday. I called it "her mature look that she sometimes has," and he nodded immediately; he knew what I meant. The sloping grave cheeks, the head held high on the sweet little neck that curves in just where you want to kiss her, and I forgot to mention the little downturned rosebudy mouth, downturned with what I call her pout-dimples, very haughty. Yes it is altogether a very haughty and wonderful, unconscious little mature look she has, and I love it. I kiss it and I treasure it with all my heart; it is so independent of me, and so *hers*. It knows life is a very grave situation and it says, "I don't care; I'm going to be all right. I'm going to march through it anyway, with my head up."

Later. The sun came out.

Today after the bread baking and during the making of the blueberry-lemon cake whose recipe Esther and I got from G, Esther took a wooden bowl of fresh blueberries out on the doorstep to eat with her hands. Her hands — chubby and graceful, pudgy and exquisite; the flesh on the little bones is plump and elastic and vigorous with young life, but the little bones inside it are quick as birds. Grubbing the blueberries with those darling hands, she was a picture. I had put the blueberry cakes in the oven to bake, and, tired after a day of baking (oh lovely day of flour going everywhere — Esther sprinkling flour on her little dough characters ... had flopped upside-down on the day-bed in the kitchen where through two open doors to and from the porch, I could see her sitting on the red wooden step, her lime-green dress — the colour looks so wild and green on her — her golden hair twisted and wound and kept up on her head to keep stray hairs out of the baking, showing the divinely-wrought little shape of her proud head, the sunshine gleaming on the burnished coils of her braid, those plump and bird-quick hands first taking the berries one by one, then grabbing handfuls and stuffing them in that pretty little mouth and chomping on them unaware that she was watched; instinctively, like an animal, a bear cub in the woods, stuffed them ... I laughed as silently as I could. She was sitting three-quarters turned away from me; behind her, our cut birch woodpile, and the tops of cherry, fir, spruce and juniper behind that. This, to answer my lovely Elliott Merrick's kind question, is how come I live in the woods.

Part 2
A Woman's Guide to Snaring Rabbits

Audubon bird count
Christmas 1993
Golden Bay
Cape St. Mary's to Point Lance
       —two bald eagles
       —three great cormorants ("shags on shag rock" — H)
       —eiders
       —two ravens
       —loon with red necked grebe
       —flock of redpolls
       —red-breasted nuthatch
       —boreal chickadee
       —flock of black scoters with oldsquaws
       —nine harlequin ducks — lords and ladies

January 16, 1994

Rabbit snaring details:

H: Build archways. The marsh looks rabbitish (behind Butterpot House). Make the sides of the snare look like under-
growth (fix boughs at each side). Drape snare area with
hay. Rabbits can smell hay. This is where a rabbit path
goes (moss indented, in a line ... also green rushes with
white pith, eaten). You can look for buttons but you don't
need to. Put the snare this high from the ground (four
fingers). They like little archways (made of boughs). You
choose a stick, tie your wire around it so it eats into the
bark, and you plunge the stick with the snare on it into the
mossy ground at an angle.

G: You won't catch rabbits on a warm night. You catch them
on a cold night because they keep moving and they move
fast. I go in on the marsh. I stick boughs on either side so
they won't go round the snare.

P: Have your snare four fingers up from the ground. Bend
your thumb and measure it.

H: Sometimes you can put two piles of birch around your
snare.

K: In Labrador rabbits eat willows. We make pounds for them
with willows inside and a space in each wall to hang your
snares.

H: Don't listen to anything he says. With pounds you have to
make a lot of them.

My father: I'll send you a pair of snowshoes. Don't cut the
straps. You need them long.

H: You can't miss a rabbit track; it's three, three, three.

G: To make pounds, stick boughs into the snow in a circle measuring five feet in diameter, with three alleys in which you place snares. Put sections of a birch tree inside the circle. The rabbits won't jump over the boughs. Or if they do, they'll go through the alleys on their way out. (The rabbits like the birch.)

When the marsh is frozen over, the rabbits travel over it.

E: This time of year I would make pounds. I would make a frame, four-sided or triangular, or octagonal, out of cut wood that had no boughs; out of sticks; about this high (almost to his knee). I would make it about five feet in diameter, and hang three or four snares. If there's something natural to hang your snare from, so much the better.

Block off your frame with boughs all around, leaving openings where the snares are. To ensure that a new snowfall won't close off your snares, make canopies or umbrellas over them with boughs.

Inside the pound, place your clusters of birch. What you want is young tips. About sixteen inches from your snare, inside the pound, place a few birch tips with the tips facing the snare, to entice the rabbit. There you have your pound.

When there is little snow, and when there is a lot of snow, are your two difficult conditions for getting rabbits. With little snow they have plenty of uncovered grasses to eat. With lots of snow they can more easily reach the tender birch tips. With a moderate amount of snow that covers the earth but does not make for easy access to the tips of branches, you will more easily entice a rabbit in this way.

I once knew a man who said he used a puncheon to trap rabbits. He'd shave the lid and attach it with a pivot to the top, place the puncheon in the snow, bank it up with snow, and place his birch cluster in the centre of the lid. The rabbit would come to eat it, and the lid would swivel, and the man would catch three or four rabbits in his puncheon this way. I don't know if he was pulling my leg.

How would you kill a rabbit (in the puncheon or in a snare)? There are several ways. You can pinch the heart. You feel it beating just above the rib-cage, and pinch it gently with your thumb and forefinger, like this; (he illustrates on Esther's purple dinosaur, a tough pinch, repeated about three times). That's the quickest way and perhaps the most humane.

Some people take the rabbit's hind legs, stretch it away from the snare, and give it a chop right behind the ears with the side of the palm. This severs the spinal cord, but there might be blood. I generally pinch the heart.

January 16, 1994

Well, I have gradually set more snares in the woods at the foot of Butterpot Mountain. So now I have ten set. Before the snow fell, I found nice rabbit paths in two places; the moss was indented in a line, and there were nice moist rabbit buttons to prove the indentations had not been made by squirrels. H and N say squirrels' paths look like rabbit paths, but only rabbits make the buttons.) I set four snares in these places.

Snow came and for awhile I kept my original snares. I would have to raise or lower them according to how much snow had fallen or melted. If I made boot-holes in deep snow I'd fill them in. H says this was right.

I saw that the rabbit tracks were in the vicinity of the summer paths I had found but did not follow them exactly, and I made new snares. At first I think my snares were too out in the open. I began to put snares in places where rabbits had gone through narrower openings in among the boughs, and my original snares I tried to made more hidden, by shrouding them with boughs.

After awhile I began to notice that I was starting to see "rabbit stories," things the rabbits had done, sequences of events, turnarounds and gathering places, nibbled willows and drinking holes. At one point, as I surveyed a place where rabbit tracks in the snow showed apparent passage through, I noticed the tracks did not continue into the woods, but centred around some pliant willows, pieces of which had fallen on the snow's crust during the repast.

In some places a lone rabbit had passed through once, but in others, such as near a cut birch by a spring, a maze of tracks circled about in what I called the rabbits' bus-stop.

Gradually I set snares in archways or enclosed passages through which I could see that numerous rabbits — or the same rabbit numerous times — had passed.

So far I have not snared a rabbit, although in my earlier

days when my snares were more visible and too large, tracks and buttons showed that rabbits had come to within an inch or two of my snares, and had decided not to go through with it. More and more I am thinking about constructing one of the "pounds." My snowshoes have arrived, a present from my father, who made them, and the marsh is frozen over now. Jim says three skidoos went passing over it yesterday evening. Maybe I will make my pound "in on the mash."

Thinking about each of my snares in turn is a relaxing way to go to sleep at night. I imagine each one, nestled in its green and snowy place. I will perhaps outline them in a future entry.

January 29, 1994

I am sitting reading *A Wreath of Roses* at DL Cafe, two cleaned and skinned rabbits beside me on the bench. B tells me he saw a special on TV on how to snare rabbits. He remembers something no one has told me yet. When you are blocking off the rabbit path with branches, you should use dry, old, scentless twigs; not new green boughs. This is because rabbits will slow down to scent, investigate and nibble new green twigs, and so will be a lot less likely to plunge through one's snare.

Found the poem, "The Rabbit Catcher" by Sylvia Plath, on the living room floor today while I was cleaning up.

B also told me it's easy to let rabbits dry out when you are cooking them, because they possess so very little body fat. So keep the lid on and do it tenderly.

I went to town yesterday so didn't check my snares. Today is pouring rain. I have twenty-one snares out now. Sometime I want to outline here each snare; its character and situation — they are very peaceful; rabbits do choose the most enchanted parts of the wood in which to run about.

Yesterday morning I saw, as H says, "how rabbits are bought and sold." We went to the loading area back of Murphy's store on Rawlin's Cross. We transferred eleven frozen rabbits with their skins still on from a cooler to a cardboard box. Murphy's gave H $10.00 a brace (pair) and H threw the eleventh rabbit in free. Murphy said he'd buy as many rabbits as H could bring.

"I'm getting away from selling them now," H said. "They're too scarce."

February 6, 1994

H: The reason rabbits are scarce is because the provincial government, in its wisdom, prohibited the hunting of lynx, forgetting that the lynx had to eat something. Foxes are getting rabbits too.

What we have here are hares, not rabbits. They aren't born in a burrow. First they huddle together but when they're a few days old they start to leave the huddle and spread out on their own, as far from the others as that truck over there, say. But if a lynx comes on the scene they run right back to their huddle very quickly, and the whole works of them are just a mouthful for the lynx.

"The Snare" (J. Stephens, from *Palgrave's Golden Treasury*)

> I hear a sudden cry of pain!
> There is a rabbit in a snare:
> Now I hear the cry again,
> But I cannot tell from where.
>
> But I cannot tell from where
> He is calling out for aid!
> Crying on the frightened air,
> Making everything afraid!
>
> Making everything afraid!
> Wrinkling up his little face!
> As he cries again for aid;
> —And I cannot find the place!
>
> And I cannot find the place
> where his paw is in the snare!
> Little one! Oh little one!
> I am searching everywhere!

The first verse of this song was written in the woods after checking my snares. No rabbits, but this song, written on a matchbook.

Bird in the Sun

> Love flies where it flies;
> You cannot devise
> a bed for love to sleep.
> Bird in the sun
> whose transparent wing
> glides on harbours deep —
> whose golden song
> ascending long

at early morning's knee
fills the wood
with ancient sound
her own heart's ease to keep.

Love woos where she woos —
no one can choose
the land where she will lie;
among slim reeds
by an unknown stream
where scraps of moonlight glide.
Her tremolo tune
hangs near the wild moon
in the dog-rose scented night —
a dream escaped
from its dreamer, dreaming
of love's immortal flight.

W: This was a good summer for the rabbits — a good year for breeding. Dry. It meant the little holes in the marshes where they breed — their burrows like — didn't fill up with water and kill off the litters.

K: Don't rabbits pick nice places for their runs?

W: (Lights up) Yeah — *cozy*, like!

Part III:
White Ptarmigan
or The Circle of Perpetual Apparition

February 12, 1994

Jim deathly sick with Bejing flu. Water still frozen and I am carrying buckets from the well.

Today tried to overcome those things with miraculous little pleasures, which see below:

Miraculous little pleasure number one: I told Esther to come and sleep with me if she woke up in the night, instead of downstairs with daddy because he was so sick. So she did. In the morning sun she was like a little bowl of trifle, just as creamy and the same colours. Her cheeks were the cream, the roses on them were the jelly, and her little pink wet tongue was the soaked cake. Her eyes were berries, and her goldy hair was chocolate sprinkles.

Two: Esther and I halved cold oranges straight from the refrigerator and I taught her to eat them the way I used to when I was little.

Three: She suggested we take ice cream to the pond for a picnic. It sure didn't melt on the way. We sat on white snowpiles on the pondside and Esther said we were in the sky, eating ice cream on the clouds. We lay on the clouds and the sun blazed down on us. A group of people with wagging dogs came past us on a skidoo, pulling a child's red toboggan that had an old man sitting on it. He was wearing a grey toque and laughing. We walked across the pond and Esther played at being one of the wagging dogs, on all fours.

Four: Even though I had to hack the well ice with the potato grubber and carry in buckets of water, I was able to see, as I cannot see when water runs through the taps, how sacred and precious it is. Taking it out of a bucket with a dipper and then pouring it is a sacred act.

Friday, February 18, 1994

There is a certain flowering magic — a euphoria — that a woman has, that she gets herself into, through a lot of inner work and intuitive floating, and that a man comes into the room, spies, and attempts to destroy, no destroys, in one violent swipe.

February 26, 1994

Profoundly exhausted and emotionally drained — body filled with emotional poisons and rage over the sickness energy pervading the house. Negativity, blame and unforgiveness. Stresses and tensions in my lower back, throat, shoulders.

A couple of people have suggested that I should be "used to it" by now — as if I should shut up about it and act as if it isn't happening. Not that I talk about it very much.

I can't take another twenty minutes of this, let alone years. It is threatening my physical health. Sometimes I think I will be the one to die of cancer. Poisoned energy is seeping. It is seeping, all through the house. This is going to go on until I am destroyed too.

The window of this juniper-loft is open. Soft night breezes are rolling in, over the backs of the stars. This rough, crumpled old notebook is coming to an end and I will have to find another.

I can hear the river gushing again, after weeks of its being frozen. The cool breeze is healing on my face and hands as I lie near the open window. H and N caught two white ptarmigans in the snares, baited with birch. H says they make good eating but he regrets having killed them. The other night I told Esther a story called "White Ptarmigan in the Snow." I told her about the two in the snares and she pouted and said they were too beautiful to kill.

I stood one day on the beach with H: waves hurled spray toward us. His weathered face was hit by the sea. Thousands of pounds of red kelp had been flung on the stones. While we were on the beach he found a little bull-bird. "Look," he said, "they are so close to the edge during the winter that any slight thing can make them perish." He placed the little bird, still alive and quivering, in the pocket of his soft, warm caramel-brown coat, and when we got back to the neat little house he put it in a box with soft cloths over and under it. I saw him cup the bird in his hands and put it to his mouth several times, to kiss it and blow warm air on it.

Friday, 4 March, 1994

Esther stayed up late lying down watching a movie with me tonight and her midnight sleepiness made her just like pounds and pounds of roses in my arms.

Have to decide whether to stay project (script) 'til September or try to have it all done by the first of May. I don't want to rush it because I feel worn out and weary, from cancer, from parenting, and from housework and money-earning responsibilities. So I do as I tell others in my journal writing class, and do a non-dominant hand dialogue:

Right Hand: What do you really want to do?

Left Hand: Rest. Art.

RH: What about fear of not having any money?

LH: You could do the work gradually and pay yourself part-time until September. That way you could keep your hand in at other stuff too; painting, encyclopedia, journalism features, teaching. Also you could accumulate more richness within and for the project by allowing it to happen over more time. Jim is sick now.

RH: Okay I'll try. And while I'm at it, I won't take on any new projects. Right?

LH: Okay.

RH: You still feel uneasy.

LH: You bet I do. I don't trust you to take care of me. Don't take on any more projects from other people's heads, and stop doing things just for the money.

RH: What heart-project have you got going that I should be devoting precious time to?

LH: Go swimming. Sauna. Go to hear the Prodigal Daughters sing. See the Piano movie. Have fun. Go see some white ptarmigans with H. Paint them. Write songs about them. Live from the heart God gave you.

RH: What about the roof, the cats?

LH: Get tar. It's cheap. Find out who wants the cat.

RH: I love you.

LH: I love you too.

March 5, 1994

My brother Paul phoned. I didn't go into any detail but when he asked how things were going I couldn't answer him and started to cry. These are some of the things he said to me:

1. It will pass. Good times will come again one day. Some people have miserable times the whole of their lives. But you're going to have a nice life when this is over. In twenty years look how things could be.

2. No, to drive over a cliff is the way to rob; rob your brothers, your parents, your daughter.

3. Don't be too hard on yourself. Remember you are not like anybody else. You are different. You were brought up different, you were born different. If anybody, your friends, anybody — tries to make you be like other people, tell them to get lost.

4. The only thing you have to do is ... ha, you don't have to do anything. There's only two things that have to happen; you have to die, and you have to pay taxes or you'll go to jail. Other than these two things, you don't have to do anything. You need to just do nothing, rest yourself. If anybody, friends, try to make you do something you don't want to do, tell them to go to hell.

5. The last thing you need is anybody trying to manipulate you. Things are bad enough without that. Life isn't easy. You have to scratch and claw and fight. If someone's giving you a hard time while you're doing that, sometimes you need to give them a good push.

6. Have a little goal every day, to help you stick it out —

if you decide to try and stick it out. You have to keep fighting. You feel like you're down in a valley and you look up and you see you've got to go all the way up that hill, and when you get to the top, there's another valley, and it keeps happening. But then there's a time when you reach a peak where you can do a few things, plant a vegetable garden. And you can stay there awhile.

Paul was comforting because he's had a hard life and he's so basic, and I loved it when he said I didn't have to do anything. I'm so wearied with people demanding and not appreciating the million and seven things I do.

March 6, 1994

My little goal today is part of "The Outlaw's Quest" discussed in my journal workshop. It is to go in on the Blue Fin* Barrens and find the beautiful White Ptarmigan. I have triple socks, roof tar on the crack in my boots where I cut the instep chopping birch with the axe H sharpened, a bag of apricots, and binoculars. It is snowing on the hills. Maybe I will never come back. (I'll get another coffee before I go.)

I told Paul I wanted to find white ptarmigan. He said they are in the tuckamoor where the barrens are, in between the barrens and woods. He said if I had a little 410 shotgun I could shoot one. He says you step on the wings, pull the feet, and the skin just comes off. I told him H got some in rabbit snares

---

* The Blue Fin was a truck-stop on the TCH in the barrens.

he had laced with birch, and he said yes. I think Valda* just wants to see the beautiful white ptarmigan, and leave it alive. I wanted to see H today, but I have to go it alone, and that's okay. My journal is good company. At the Blue Fin, with a coffee, the endless barrens rolling out the wide windows, and the snow.

Consolations:

— Strengthening my options:

> White ptarmigan
> Rabbits
> Learning about wilderness
> Swimming
> I can get away, for spells.

— Myself: Always I have myself.

I wouldn't mind just going on trips in the country with H now — seeing wild creatures in their homes, having a laugh, listening to him talk in his low, dark voice like black cake and brandy, or just walking together, on foot or on snowshoes or on skis — fishing together, lying under the stars. I love the way he makes toast and tea on a fire, the wild, energetic way he strides over the wild heath or the parking lot.

I'll go out now, into the wild black and white landscape,

---

* Valda was a comic-book woman hero in papers KW's grandfather sent her when she was a child. To restore her vitality before a new adventure, Valda would step into a cold blue fire and emerge totally re-energized. KW remembers Valda and identifies with her here and at other times in her life.

under which lies the warm barrens, where the white ptarmigan shelters and flies.

A few hours later:

Behind the Blue Fin past boulders much larger than the many junipers. Straw-coloured pitcher plant skeletons showing through the crust of snow — also wild rhododendron and star-moss. Glad I had my snowshoes. Climbed an enticing mountain then sat on my snowshoes on lee of topmost boulder, and looked through binoculars (Paul's) for caribou and ptarmigan, but saw none. Heard the "speeph" of soft waves of hard snow sweeping on the mountain's snow-crust.

If I saw no ptarmigan still I was on ptarmigans' land, and breathed the air they have breathed, touched what they have touched, and maybe next time I will see one. Checked tuckamoor, juniper and birch shelters for ptarmigan. Saw tracks of what may have been a lynx. Thinking of future outings; with Esther to Cape St. Francis — with H to Cape Spear. I would like to see more owls, eagles, ptarmigan, caribou and moose; wild birds flying alone, wild geese flying together, like I saw on the pond as I sat alone making a watercolour.

Later:

Phoned H: He and Nathaniel saw 35 or 40 white ptarmigans in the snow last Thursday. They were on the barrens, on a flat white expanse that had "some kind of stems" about two feet long emerging from the snow. They were near the shelter of a thicket of trees, with a river running through — "The perfect place for them," H said.

Little goals. My little goal yesterday was to check out the CBS swimming pool. It's a beautiful pool — with a round, shallow pool Esther will love — a whirlpool with painted palm trees, and a sauna. My Piscean body revelled in it — doing laps, then sweltering in the hot tub and sauna, then more laps, then a shower —the place so clean and beautiful.

Today my little goal was to see the exhibit of paintings of waterfowl at MUN gallery — there were a number of paintings of harlequins — mostly the paintings were done in opaque gouache or oils — but some had watercolour backgrounds, and one (geese) was done entirely in transparent watercolour.

H said today on the phone that the ptarmigans Nathaniel saw were lit and tinged with pink — he said they were beautiful. He said that pink light glows on them like that sometimes — and that it's something no-one ever photographs or paints. I'm supposed to be going out there tomorrow, but I may not go. If I do go, my little goal for tomorrow will be once again trying to catch a glimpse of a white ptarmigan in the snow.

Yesterday I cleaned the chimney and patched the roof. Much rain tonight and none coming down in the house. It surprised me that the breaks in the roof coincide exactly with where we had leaks. I was expecting it to be more complicated than that.

Also yesterday I saw a black-backed woodpecker chipping bark off a dying spruce tree, on my walk in past Butterpot Pond.

James heard snipe winnowing the other night. The following night (on my way out to go swimming) I heard it too — over the marsh, in the mass of cold stars — a lonely, thrilling sound. It's early for snipe. H said, "Where'd they find a bit of water now?"

My book says the winnowing sound is made by their tails as they hurtle from great heights in darkness or on overcast days during spring "courtship."

Esther, James and I heard new bird songs the past couple of mornings.

It seems the woodpecker, snipes, and morning songbirds have proclaimed spring is here before any of us out-of-touch humans appeared to know it. I feel it though. I felt it as soon as the winter solstice came; felt the sap rising in the birches.

Tonight Jim said think how lonely a grave is, always out there in the rain, in any weather, while people have parties and do other warm things; a grave is always lonely. I asked him if he was afraid of the loneliness of his own grave, and he said yes. He coughs and looks very dejected and sick. He talked about the "day of the dead" celebrated in Mexico, when people have big parties in graveyards, and even bring skeletons home for the festivities. "It's great," he said.

We seemed to get along okay, a bit easier, tonight. He says that's because I'm escaping to the valley of diamonds in the morning.

Wednesday, March 9, 1994

A cup of tea.

> (Trying to let pass Jim's continual comments about
> how I am the most selfish, evil and inconsiderate
> person in the universe. Trying to at least let one
> person's life be cheerful: mine.)

My day down in the valley of diamonds: The sea was
green and purple. In it the Virgin Rocks (upon which H has
lain and duck-hunted) lay luminous pale blue, with shim-
mering silver hollows. Waves billowed toward the shore
flinging behind them joyful vapours of spume — sea horses.
H took me "tromping around." First we went to the valley of
diamonds, through moose dens and lacy rabbit gates (they'll
choose a tidy one every time, H says), and trees whose
curvature rivals lilac and monkey-puzzles; to a bluff over-
looking this valley of diamonds, so named for reasons unknown and mysterious. A seal rookery lay below. Then we
went to a special meadow where in summer the heath is
covered in bluebells. Today spray was being blown up over
the heath from a waterfall below on the cliff face; we ran
through the glorious spray, which had covered all the little
heath plants in a coat of silver ice. We saw fox tracks and
tromped through H's mother's bakeapple berry picking
grounds. A seal rookery lay below this place too. H says they
have their babies in March, and they lie on the rocks sunning
themselves in summer; he has gone up to them in a dory and
touched them.

Having a little goal each day is really worth it. One thing

I would like to do soon is go to St. Michael's, visit Mrs. Tee's grave, and find out what seabird life is happening there around the islands now. Another thing I'd like to do is see which birds are flying north past Cape Race. I'd also like to visit Cape St. Francis. For tomorrow I may have a look at where the osprey's nest was last year, and see if there's any springtime osprey activity there again this year.

Thursday, March 10, 1994

At a coffee shop after teaching my journal writing class. Mourning the lost apparition, mirage, illusion, of love. I make myself subservient to wisdom, and what is wisdom's reward? Suffering. (I am wishing for the mirage, the fata morgana. Fata morgana is what the Virgin Rocks were like — castles in the air.)

Today there were two "little goals" — I walked to where the ospreys' built their nest last year. I knew the old nest had blown down. I went to see if there was any sign of new nest-making. There wasn't, but the trip was, of course, not wasted: I walked up the hill through the woods to the transmission line, and found a large rock wreathed in tangled deadwood on which to sit. To sit I had to turn and face the direction from which I'd come, and the colour made me gasp. On the way up it had been all browns, greens, and the watery white of melting snow: when I turned I saw the distant mountains were covered in blue — dark blue — energy. I felt the energy of the spring earth, air and water; the immense energy that is in everything at all times; strong and burgeoning now, in early spring; later, in summer, all expanded and effervescent.

Took James along the Witless Bay Line to St. Michael's to feel some of that island sea energy. (The girl in here is stacking the chairs and tables and sweeping the floor.)

March 16, 1994

Snipe Winnow
I hear the rushing river
... and over it, the snipe's haunting lament
winnowing over the marsh
at midnight in the fog.

The snipe's winnow is the marsh's secret
behind spring's unlocking
of pitcher plant leaves
star mosses
wine-filled marshberries
pungent gin-berries
soft, orange-centred haws
smell of snow melting
and the black peat softening

Rabbit tracks in the woods trails
their getaways graceful and tidy
and tracks of little squirrel feet —
large tracks where a moose crossed
and broke through the snow on the marsh
— the water frozen where it seeped up
— little belly-hair curl marks
where the moose faltered in the snow
and on the little paths
lithe, quick grosbeaks,

chartreuse female and dried raspberry male
clicking larch buds,
a multitude of husks floating on the snow

Pure streams flow from the mountain
whose face I have seen blue and topped
with the year's first snow
under a white full moon,
whose brow I have seen crowned
with gold junipers under a moon gold as goldenrod —
Now the melted snow flows pure for drinking

and the snipe's winnow
haunts the marsh
being the sound of the marsh's soul,
lonely like all souls

March 21, 1994. Spring Equinox.

Apparently the sun "crossed the line" at 5 p.m. yesterday, at
which time I was rambling in solitude over the barrens,
marshes and woodland trails, under a sky full of gold and
pink clouds. I heard a "whirr" under the bushes lining the
transmission line — could it have been a Spring Equinox
ptarmigan sounding the song of its changing colours?
Chewed a refreshing leaf of Indian Tea plant, inhaling the
fragrance of a sprig I carried crushed in one hand, as I
clambered the golden hills lined underneath the gold with
new fern greens, mosses and rubies of wild rhododendron
and Sarracenia purpurea.

For several days (amidst conflicts and the old discom-
forts) I have felt tenderness for my little family, Jim and
Esther, and incredible love for our little home — which Jim

says is like a gypsy caravan under the stars, the rushing river and winnowing snipe a spiralling song around our little tent. I would like to get some shingles and paint out of the money for the new script; Egyptian rose (gold rose, the colour of Egypt or the Spring Equinox clouds) for the bathroom, and midnight blue for the outside, with lemon cream sashes.

Later: After talking to H:

Told H about the whirring bird sound I heard in the underbrush — he made the sound exactly over the phone — he said it was a grouse disturbed by my coming close.

25 March, 1994

Saw a female black-backed woodpecker in the trail beyond the shacks toward the transmission line. It was drumming at a dead spruce. It was definitely black-backed. I had binoculars. Uncommon according to my Golden "Birds of North American" — here is what it says:

> "Black-backed woodpecker (Picoides arctus)
> Uncommon even in its preferred habitat — dead conifers, from which it peels bark. Note barred sides and black back. (I did -kw) In East, only this and the much larger Pileated have solid black backs. In West only Lewis' and White-headed have black back and rump. Only the male has yellow crown. Call, a sharp pik."

26 March, 1994

Wild-Hearted

Now, in late March, the melted brook
candles over mossy rock into a pool
where stones await the end of the earth,
but you,
enchanted like the pool
and like the rabbits' graceful gates,
are far from me, among the trout springs
of your gold heath,
ruby berry,
eagle, duck, cormorant,
little bull-bird, sweet rabbit;
creatures safe from you,
wild and shy as you are,
though you are brown with the sun's courage,
swift with running in the woods,
far-sighted with looking on the sea,
wild-hearted with the wind's freedom.

28 March, 1994

"Therefore the flight shall perish from the swift, and
the strong shall not strengthen his force, neither shall
the mighty deliver himself:
Neither shall he stand that handles the bow; and he
that is swift of foot shall not deliver himself: neither
shall he that rides the horse deliver himself.
And he that is courageous among the mighty shall
flee away naked in that day, says the Lord."

Amos 2:14-16

but "He fails not."

Zephan iah 3:5.

29 March, 1994

"And Saul was afraid of David, because the Lord was
with him, and was departed from Saul."
1 Samuel 18:12

My soul is no longer downcast — it is filled with anticipation
and happiness and creative energy over this new script project — which just goes to reinforce what I try to remind myself
is true — keep creative and your soul will not be downcast for
long. Before the script meeting I took myself for a good walk
through the woods and along the transmission line — got a
good lot of icy marsh-water in my boot, sat down on a
sunwarmed bit of moss and looked upon the distant hills for
a good while, with my binoculars.

April 8, 1994

North West River, Labrador

I am speechless at this land; it speaks to my heart. Two
nights ago Janet and I stood on the ice off North West River
beach and watched my first display of Northern Lights. I
cannot speak adequately to reveal how this land, ice and sky
speak to me. North West River is like New Mexico in its big
spaces/sky, distant mountains, and sunlit buildings like the
Northern store with its mix of Innu and Metis and white
settlers.

North West River has water all around it, in distinct kinds
of geography; the south side of Hamilton Inlet with its lining
of mystery-blue, snow-dusted mountains leading out to the
sea; the narrowing rapids leading on into the mighty Grand

Lake and Beaver, Susan and Naskapi rivers; and Mokami Mountain, and Mulligan and the islands on the north side of Lake Melville.

The town of North West River is ever so pretty, and the crescent beach that sweeps behind this point where the Bs live has sand that T says the kids used to call sugar. The sand has dune grasses that now stick out of the snow. The trees of this area are much, much taller than the houses, and dark and straight and symmetrical. Their boughs have spaces between and match up on each side beautifully. Wind sighs through these tall trees, and rattles and whispers through the beach grass.

The buildings are often low houses, with windows that have many panes, old-fashioned and very inviting in the snow, with the dark spruce and clean drifts. Sparkling little homes, some of which have snowshoes hung outside the doors, and woodsmoke softly coming out of the chimneys. Most have skidoos and komatiks by the front, and boats and kin-oos (canoes) sheltered in the boughs of spruce sheltering the gardens. Today with Janet and her neighbour Judy, I went to the Northern store and the craft store. I got a little doll for Esther, made in Sheshatshit; a child swaddled and laced up with a rawhide thong — a sweet little thing — and I got her a soft white rabbit-skin too. Janet offered to teach me how to make moccasins, so I bought some skin and grey rabbit fur and three square-topped needles, and I plan to go across to her house tomorrow, Saturday. How nice of her to offer to teach me.

Her patterns, for different sizes of moccasins and different styles — gathered, or the type called "rabbit nose" — are made out of newspaper and brown paper, and were bequeathed to her by her husband's mother.

Harry Martin is launching his new recording at a concert in Goose Bay tomorrow, and T was able to get me a ticket. His neighbour M will take me if it's not too stormy. To hear Harry Martin will be a thrill.

I love North West River. It stirs my heart. T and Janet are beautiful, true souls. It really means something for me to be here.

July 23, 1994

Today Esther and I gathered masses of wild rose petals and I made my wild rose and rhubarb jam (into which this year I also poured a bowl of Butterpot Road wild strawberries), as well as a rhubarb rose petal pie now chilling in the refrigerator.

We are broke but the nasturtiums are out. Tonight as I cut up tinned tomatoes over soaking navy beans for tomorrow, Jim was saying Dr. Ganguly said, "When the obstruction starts, you may last three months, or only a few weeks." Jim feels this obstruction on his heart. He has palpitations of the heart and fears he may be dying. Each other year of his cancer he has said, "Well, I may make it to Christmas," because he loves Christmas. But this summer he has been telling people he may die in the fall.

As I cut through the soft tomatoes some tears gushed out

and my mouth went all upside down like Esther's crying. Jim said, "Don't cry into the beans," and then he came up with a little gray stone to which he'd affixed a blob of chewed bubblegum inside its wrapper.

"Don't cry, ma cherie," said the little stone. It was Maurice Chevalier. He (Maurice) is up in the kitchen cupboard now.

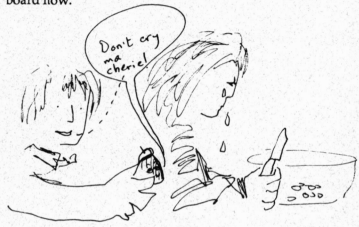

Saturday, July 30, 1994

Today was a blessed day from the beginning; rain had showered the night and by morning sunshine came out and twinkled all the wild roses and fairy grasses; the humid oppression of yesterday washed away.

Put a white chair in the green bower or fairy glade and sat

there alone, then with Esther, then got Jim to sit there and he loved it too, in the filtered birch-leaf light. Then J and B came with their beautiful children, and we had an afternoon together, during which E and his daughter brought the brown hen I'd asked for. This evening I worked more on constructing hen house. A hen is a blessed thing — eggs — brown eggs — from heaven, Jim says. She laid us an egg on the way here.

August 6, 1994

Just to record a dream I had last night: B and I were in a clearing in the woods where I was showing her a really nice junkyard with an antique couch and some chairs and things that had once been beautiful and were now of dubious value even to us. It felt as if we might find something wonderful if we looked long enough, but it was possible we'd only find things useless with all their beauty dissolved out of them with time and the rain in the woods.

At first things seemed laid in a disorderly way, then as we proceeded through the stuff it became more ordered. We came to a long narrow shack and went in; the junk had been leading to it, and the junk continued inside it; somewhat disorderly in the first room, but more carefully arranged as we proceeded into another room, then another. This third room was a kitchen, and for the first time I felt someone lived here. Alarmed, I went to a dark hallway leading to more rooms, and bumped into a middle-aged woman, who wore a bathrobe and carried a large mesh bag full of shining white creatures.

"Oh, I'm sorry," I said. "We didn't realize anyone lived here."

"That's all right," she told us, "you're just in time for supper." Out of the sack she took a white creature. It was some kind of fish; fat, with white "frills" along it, and very solid and lithe. It flipped from her hands and landed back in her hands. She said it was a salamander — the bag was full of salamanders. She said they were easy to catch — they just crawled in under her door. She held the salamander in her arms — it seemed very big — then she cleaned it and took something out of its insides and cleaned and cut the remaining flesh, which was thin and flat like leather.

Meanwhile she had B eating a bowl of salamander soup. B put a spoonful to my lips, which I did not appreciate. But, not wanting to offend the woman, I ate it. The piece of salamander was slippery and chewy like squid. So the woman, who had short sandy brown hair, cooked her flat pieces of salamander flesh in a pan of oil. "See how they float in the oil as they roast," she said. She said you could fry them as well as roast them, but she liked them roasted. I wondered if she called it roasting because she was using oil and not hard fat. We ate the salamander, cutting squares of it like you would cut pancakes, and it was mild-tasting and chewy. That was the end of the dream.

I think I dreamed it because we don't have any money. Obviously she didn't either. Even though the salamander tasted okay, I felt pretty yucky about it; it "crawled" under her door, and then there was all this junk everywhere, like the old seat on our deck. Our house is still half-painted, although progress has been made, and the stone walkway is half done, and then there's my makeshift scrap wood chicken coop, and Esther's plastic wading pool in the yard. It's all so poor and pathetic, especially when I have no money coming in, and little self esteem because of it. I guess I feel something like the woman — getting older in the middle of a pile of ruined stuff, living on what I can manage to scrounge — her being in her bathrobe at supper time was just another sign of poverty and unemployment.

I got up and took the rug off the deck rail where I washed it and left it hanging too long so it got musty. It's hot and humid outside, and I feel disgusted about having no money; I feel poor and worthless.

August 12, 1994

Today the hospital phoned and asked for Jim to go in for chemical treatment. I don't like calling it chemotherapy or especially "chemo" because it sounds gentle, even affectionate, and I figure it's a no-win situation — poisonous chemicals causing nausea, hair fallout and death. But I see now Jim will die without it sooner probably, because the constriction in his throat means he can't breathe or swallow freely.

Fifteen hundred dollars came in the mail the day after the salamander dream, from CBC and from Peter Gzowski.

Koosy is laying an egg every day.

I've been crying a lot in comparison with how much I've cried over the cancer in the past two years — or crying for a different reason — I just feel sad, very sad about Jim. For once in my journal I can't translate into words how I feel, except in this simplest, most basic, childlike of ways — I'm sad. Sad and crying.

Today he wore a light blue shirt and dark trousers and his grey jacket. The outfit lit up the blue of his eyes. His face isn't puffy now because of the change from the $10.00 steroids to the $170.00 steroids. He was saying this past few days, with the comfort the new medication brought him, was an oasis — things would never be the same after the call to go in for the chemical treatment. If they give him the really strong kind then his hair will fall out. Esther and I took him to the Health Sciences Centre. We waited in the admitting area, then took him to his room, which looked like somebody's workshop, or a warehouse. A couple of old men lay in beds on one side. On the other side near the door was Jim's narrow, high, hard-looking "bed." In the corner a large space was devoted to piles of boxes containing oxygen tubes, masks and other paraphernalia. There was a sweet, gut-wrenching hospital stench in the room. They told him on the phone he would be in there two days, but the form the nurse had said five. Esther cried when we were to leave, and held onto him and said she would miss him. They had a long, loving, silent hug, him sitting on his bed, her huggling into him. I went to see B after. I told her I felt sad. I told her I felt my little world is being pulled apart. She cried with me and said, "I know, and it's such a beautiful one too."

B said she's glad I'm able to be with Jim now, that I never

left him. I'm glad now too. Every day I'm glad over it. Jim and I laughed about it this morning.

August 17, 1994

One of the reasons my memory slips back into the sedateness of lives begun in 1900 — the muskmallow flower of old world gardens, the cobblestones and the rag-and-bone man — has to do with the pain of being. When everything connected with another person seems sedate, or lovely, or spiritual, or some other desirable thing — whether it is because of the time past in which they lived, or the present things with which they surround themselves — then we think that person is like those things. That is why I married my husband, I now see. Because of the lovely things with which he surrounded himself: great literature, Irish poetry, mystical Indian incense, and the lofty arches of Handel and Bach. But I now know that he is himself none of those things. If you were to put him alone in a room — marriage — and expect him to be like any of these things, you would be disappointed. For a person is not what he surrounds himself with, or what he aspires to, or longs for.

Before we were married, one day in his monk's room, surrounded by musty books which he liked to sniff, and ink bottles, and old varnished furniture and the recording of a boy soprano singing Mozart's Requiem — he unaccountably began singing "The Great Pretender."

"Oh yes, I'm the great pretender," he sang smugly, "I seem to be what I'm not, you see ..."

I have never forgotten it. How often we judge a person based on just such a veil of illusion. Which is why biographies can be so captivating; a memento here, a scrap of lace there; a remembered, wistful conversation overheard on a verandah and recorded in a diary — when the person is dead there is no one to prove that these things were just illusory shadows, and that most of them had nothing to do with who the person really was.

And who is a person, really? How do you measure and know and feel who he really is, when the projector lighting all the swimming scraps of his comfort and wistfulness and dream is turned off? For these are all things that go into the person; the things he feeds his soul. Who he really is, is what comes out of him; what his soul feeds to others. And his body too.

(A couple of days ago I really did meet a middle-aged woman with short hair who said she used to have pet salamanders.)

Sunday, August 21, 1994

The Raleigh three-speed I bought two days ago at the liquida-
tion centre — how perfect it is. I flew around the old school
road on it yesterday morning, then along Country Path Road,
where I had not been before, and where I saw a chestnut beast
of a horse that whinnied at me, his nostrils flaring in symme-
try, his muscles oiled and gleaming, his mane a wing of
freedom. I saw a grove of trembling aspen whose leaves I
heard first, like rain falling. I stopped my bike before this
grove and bared the back of my neck to the cool breeze and
rain sound. Of course I was reproached and condemned for
daring to stay out so long, but by the middle of my return
back down country path road I was doing what I used to do
all the time and never do any more, which is happily singing.

By 10:30 in the nights Jim is in bed now, following the
chemical treatments, and so is Esther. It is only when riding
my new bicycle, or reading or writing or sitting drinking tea
in this post 10:30 silence with the breezes sounding through
the trees beyond the open windows ... that I realize the
burden has not murdered my joyful spirit. I still have a joyful
spirit that can sing, and within a quarter of an hour of being
alone, my joyful spirit has fanned out her wings and is taking
pleasure in the sound and scent of a night breeze, the breathing of a lace curtain at the open window, the gold of the
lamp's light on the wood of a kitchen chair, the cool lumines-
cence of the moon in the indigo sky among the juniper-tops.

"I wish I was dead now," he said tonight, "away from
this. Away from pains and sadness."

September 2, 1994

A new book on the subject.

Well the chemical treatment has made true James' surmise that his well-being a little while ago was but an oasis — after the treatment, he said, nothing would be the same.

He has been so weak and sick and wretched that I could not leave the house for more than an hour, and lately not at all without Esther, so needless to say I have been worn out. But I prayed to God for help and in the past two weeks he has given us a lot of help, and small blessings in our midst for which I am grateful. People bare the beauty of their souls in a house of sorrow.

Poor James, I can truly pity him now.

I sit at D.L. Cafe in St. John's, Janice having gone to our house in Holyrood last night (Thursday) to stay and care for Jim and Esther until tomorrow morning, to give me some respite, which I am soaking up joyfully and gratefully.

(What horrifies me most is the smell — the smell of the stuff he is coughing up into his Great Aunt Mary-Ann's antique white chamber pot with the green roses pattern. It infiltrates the room where he is lying — his sick room — and spreads its fingers slowly throughout all the lower rooms of the house. "I hate the smell, but I love Daddy." — Esther.)

(I have to go on more about the smell:)

The first morning that it was really bad — the morning after I persuaded him to take a warm bath

(His thin legs,
stubbly chin so he wouldn't

bleed shaving because the
"chemotherapy" makes clotting
weak,
—me taking his socks off for him
—him only getting in the tub for
a minute; bubbly and very full,
the heater on in the room, a clean
purple towel
—the smell in the bathroom mixed
with the soap-fragrant steam
—clean pyjamas)
—The morning after this, I went into the sick-room and
there was a freshness there in comparison — hardly any of
the smell (which I had thought must be accumulated stuffi-
ness mixed with the sweet hospital stench which is inexplica-
ble and which nobody ever stops to analyze that I know of —
they think as I did that it is a combination of things related to
sickness, but I have found the source, and Jim said it is the
smell of Death ...)
... I went out again. Half an hour later I went back in and
the powerful stench caused me to shake from head to foot. In
the chamber-pot was a pool of greyish liquid that he had
coughed up — so it must have been the source of the smell,
and it was (is). Wherever he goes to lie down — his bed, the
daybed in the kitchen — the smell begins to curl around the
air as he coughs, as he breathes, and it wrenches right to my
stomach, it is so powerful.
I phoned the doctor to ask him what the smell could

mean (an infection) and he came and said it might be "a touch of pneumonia" or septicaemia (a septic lung). I believe it is at least a septic lung — and possibly a putrefying, decaying lung, a dead and rotting lung — with my poor Jim around it, mercilessly still alive (but not wholly mercilessly ... "touch of Jesus, spirit of Jesus ..." — Sharon)

(The doctor also perused the slip with the chemical treatments outlined on it and told Jim that compared to the next scheduled chemical (September 6th), the previous one was "nothing." This one, he said, will make you "really sick" — I reluctantly let him take the slip with the chemical names on it without writing them down first — I would like to get them from him (to make this document complete) ... This coming chemical, said the doctor, will make your hair fall out and kill the cells lining your stomach and the cells of your blood, and you will tear your guts out throwing up, and you will have no energy at all, you will be really, really sick.

So now Jim is saying he might not take the chemicals (which the doctors at the cancer clinic say have only a 30 per cent chance of shrinking — not eliminating — the throat obstructing tumour which seems to be the one that is going to kill him finally.)

"The (chemicals) do thirty things wrong and maybe only do one thing right." —Jim.)

Me and A talking about our lives:

(She is like the nasturtium vinegar I had infusing in the sunshine on the step in glass bottles the other day; glittering and sparkling and cheerful, an exquisite Egyptian Gold Rose colour ...)

How hard they have become.

I was saying that in all the many cancer books I have, there seems to be a requisite paragraph on "the caregiver." It goes something like this:

"The caregiver will sometimes experience moments of difficulty. The person with cancer may not act like his or her usual self, and patience and consideration must be exercised. Often the caregiver will feel tired. The caregiver should seek out help from cancer support groups in the community, and should take care to get sufficient rest and nourishment during the time he or she will be caring for a person with cancer."

They don't say anything about the smell. They should say something about the two friends getting together, and one asking "the caregiver" how much of the "stuff" is in the chamber pot (because her own healthy husband has just gone into the sick room and will have to face it.)

A: How much of the stuff is in it? Is it a bowl?

K: It's an old-fashioned white chamber pot with green roses on it.

A: Is it emptied out?

K: No, I didn't think to empty it out.

A: Is it deep?

K: Oh! No. I think it's only a few globs right now.... I feel awful saying this stuff to you.

A: It's all right. I can take gross. I can handle gross.

They should all put that in their "caregiver" sections.

Monday, September 5, 1994

Jim finally went to the hospital last night, at 8:30, in Hickey's ambulance.

They came to the house with flashlights and carried him to the door in a chair, and laid him in a stretcher and took him in the ambulance.

The last thing he said to Esther after she kissed him was, "Have a good time in school, Esther."

I saw the ambulance attendants give each other a look when they were helping him off the couch in the living room and he was coughing great amounts of the terrible death mucous into the plastic bag (because he was being made to move; he could not move at all without the coughing.)

The look said, He will never come back into this house again.

Me and Esther, standing on the deck. Esther up in my arms, waving gently to the illuminated glass square, the back of the ambulance, Daddy in the square on the stretcher, waving back to Esther; them taking him away.

Sharon's phone call:

The cancer doctor on call, Dr. Samanth, said it's serious. Took x-ray: said dosage of steroid decadron should be being gradually decreased. Infection could be caused by tumour, by the decadron, or by the chemotherapy (and today it will be either sunny, dull or rainy). He used the word "realistically" about four times, Sharon said. Realistically, if Jim is going to refuse more "chemotherapy" (which he told the doctor he was), then the tumour will have no choice but to grow. With the chemical treatment the tumour may subside "for the time being"

(with all the chemical
treatment's "side"-effects).

The cancer doctor understood why Jim wanted no more chemical treatment.

Realistically, he said, the place for Jim to go, if he survives this infection, is the palliative care unit at St. Clare's hospital.

While Sharon was here she brought with her the spirit of Jesus and healing for me in my relationship with Jim — I was able to forgive and love him, finally; a miracle needed at this time.

Realistically, said Dr. Samanth, patients such as James are given a "code" by the medical team at the hospital. The code means that if heart failure occurs, or any other vital function fails, the medical team will not try to revive the person.

Esther and Mommy and how Esther feels about Daddy: a drawing:

Mommy: Would you like to draw a picture about how you feel about Daddy?

Esther: Yes. I'll draw some things I want to do later with Daddy if he gets better. This is us swimming together. I have my arms around Daddy's neck. You are swimming. This is me and Daddy sitting on a grey rock, fishing.

Mommy: Do you want to draw a picture of how your heart feels?

Esther: Yes. Scrambly because I feel bad. And here's a star. I love Daddy so much.

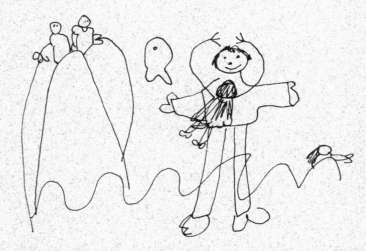

Mommy: Do you want to draw a picture of how your mind and your head feel? Do they feel anything about Daddy?

Esther: Yes, sad. Write a song about it. Can we write a song?

Daddy Stuff (a song: words by Esther)

Getting me candy
Lighting incense
Telling me stories
Going to the pond with me
And going to the grocery stores with me
Getting me kiwis
Getting me the pram
Picking wild flowers

Playing ball
Going to the park
Getting the egg
Cleaning the hen house

I love Daddy

(It's still Monday ...)
St. John's

Death
My husband's thin legs
as he lies without life
or joy or strength
in his hospital bed
—his legs, they are sad
so thin.

His hair — the portion
that he did not get me to
cut because it had
formed dead and matted
clumps; that portion is
now bare — his hair
is littering the hospital
pillow — feathery snakes
all over the plump whiteness;
or else it is clumped
and snaking, still long;
or else it has fallen
out and has left parts
of bare scalp

(His hair that once I
kissed as I said
goodbye to him on
Water Street — it
was burnished in
the setting sun,
and waving, and young

103

...His hair that once
he wore to his elbows
in a long sheen,
and was proud of
...his hair, that he
had always been
proud of...)

He said Dr. Samanth "spooked" him, talking of palliative care units, of codes, and of imminent death.

I asked a nurse how I should find out about getting help — I could not look after him at home any more.

She was surprised I was not already getting help.

The hospital usually arranges it when "the caregiver" is having trouble managing at home.

She showed me James' sheet —
"Pneumonia"

(Does he have pneumonia, I asked. They think he might, she said.)

"Consider consult
palliative care."

Are you allowed to write anything on that sheet?" I asked.

"What do you want me to write?"

"That I need to talk to someone about looking after him. Do you mean I don't have to go to social services and wait in line and see one person after another in offices and perhaps be refused help?" (This was what Dr. Walsh told me to do ...)

"No. The hospital arranges help for you at home. Would

you like me to write that you request a meeting with house staff regarding home management?"

"Yes."

So she did, and she said they will call me.

Jim said Dr. Samanth said he may not be able to go home again.

Tuesday, September 6, 1994

Tonight Esther got ready for her first day of school; tomorrow she starts kindergarten; got ready without Daddy; he must have thought about it tonight in hospital; not there for his only little one's first day of school.

Saw the doctors and social workers today — it looks as though they are prepared to help me look after him.

The disease and treatment are so degrading: the dead, matted clumps of hair which I cut for him; his bony legs like skeletons; the spitting, his utter incapacitation, lying in that bed with his legs so very thin, and just two weeks ago he was in what he called "an oasis" (before chemical treatment) ... "After that," he said then, "things are never going to be the same again."

Crayons. Scissors. Construction paper. Scrap book. Pencils. Scribblers. Pink binder. Bookbag. Bath. Pinafore dress and blouse. Shoes. Tights. Sleepyhead.

Saturday, 10 September 1994

Today Esther and I went to be with Jim at the hospital for most of the afternoon and evening. Esther was very kind and loving to him: didn't seem to mind that his hair has mostly fallen out — I told her it would be like that — kissed him and stroked his head and said he was cute. He was very moved by her love.

I told the social worker about my plans to go away for a week. I also said I did not want Jim at home unless I had some help. She said the doctors were talking about having a person from palliative care come over to consult with them and with Jim to see if he should be admitted there. The social worker had told me the doctors were saying Jim may have only "weeks" left.

Dr. Samanth said, "weeks to months, but he could surprise us all by living a couple of years." The "odour" (he is the only person who has mentioned it) has not gone, and it will take time to clear this infection, if it clears at all. "My own feeling," he said, "is that if he goes home there is a good chance he'll end up back in hospital."

He said the palliative care unit will have as its purpose "symptom control." Jim does not have to feel he's being ushered from one building to another just to die, and never see home again. Palliative care is to control (make bearable) the cancer symptoms (strangulation?) and many people visit home numerous times during their stay. I said that was important — this happened so suddenly, and Jim never got a chance to say goodbye to his home.

Doing it like that (palliative care), said the doctor, with home visits, would likely be easiest on Jim.

Jim doesn't see why he needs to go there as his pneumonia seems to be clearing up and he does not have other terrible "symptoms."

He wants me to be at the hospital with him "all the time."

He does not want me to go away next week.

He feels powerless. He feel things are beyond his control. He feels sad and lonely.

When we left to go (Esther had eaten meatballs in sauce and seasoned home fries from the cafeteria in Jim's room at suppertime) he stood up.

He was wearing new pyjamas, with little dark red diamonds on them given to him by M, and the cream-coloured fishing hat with the little brim and ludicrous loops given him by P. He put out both arms — one for me and Esther each — and hugged us.

He was very warm, and trembling ever so slightly all through and down his body, like a little bird. We left him still standing there, warm, imperceptibly but thoroughly trembling, standing straight and still, his wispy head half enclosed by the little cream brimmed hat. He had been crying, and the rims of his eyes were wet. "I'm worn out," he said, "I wish I could get better." (I sat on the bed with him and held my arm around him.)

P phoned me after I told her the doctors were talking about palliative care, and went on about bringing him home to die, honouring his wishes, etc. I defended myself more than I wished to (the smell; his slow strangulation in front of Esther; having to administer drugs and oxygen etc.; having no-one to help me ... being already worn out myself ...).

"Get all your friends and his family to do shifts," she said
—"the only thing is, *we're* very busy."

I asked my mother if she thought I was being cruel.

She said I would look back on all this and feel very sad,
but I would wonder where I had got the strength. (Not to get
drawn into the sadness; not to let it destroy me.)

D said, "There are people who'd be hanging off the
hospital bed, bawling, — they'd let it destroy them, and
they'd be no good to anyone."

A said, "Go on your week's holiday. Have a rest and
come home strong to be there for him."

Michael said, "You're doing the best you can. Above and
beyond what anyone could ask for in a relationship."

All the same, that picture of Jim as we left him (I didn't
want to cast a final glance back: it was almost as if he re-
mained standing there deliberately staring so that *I would* (I
did look back)— I could see him: a still, standing figure in that
hat, those pyjamas; whose warm, bird-trembling body I had
just held (the brim of the hat bending the tip of my right ear
down) ...

Later, tonight, I passed by the book *Dandelion Wine* in the
sickroom and recalled hearing the song by that name on Max
Ferguson: days of our Celtic youth; when we sat by the
firelight on Argyle Street (were we happy together?) listening
to the song, drinking the golden liqueur-like wine that I'd
make out of the Argyle Street dandelions of 1992 ... the
summer before we knew about the cancer ... thinking of how
it was, how we were ... that in spite of all the discord in these

diary entries we were happy together then, we did have something together; we did love each other.

I remember D coming to our lofty place on Cathedral Street one of those first Christmases (birds in a nest; goose; partridge ... on the tree) and her saying how much love and peace were in our home.

Forlorn, forsaken and afraid; trembling; warm in a cold hospital room; dying ...

A closed casket, he said today. The photo by Mannie beside it.

It seemed so sad that he was able to speak, and be Jim, and yet be so close to death; to render any time he has left futile and hopeless; as if his body had lost him, was looking for him, and could not find him ... "him" being his life. His life has been taken away from him, but he is still here, looking for it. Oh how sad.

Poor little Esther was making a grand game out of a pair of surgical gloves and the blue plastic washing-bowl near the sink. She wore a flowered sun-dress and straw hat with matching ribbon and cherries to cheer up Daddy. Victoria had given it to her. On the way to the hospital we stopped at a Marie's Mini-Mart to get a soft-serve ice-cream each; and we passed a Harley biker couple with their little girl who was all dressed in black — leotard, belt and leggings — with her hair pulled up in a rebel knot; what a photograph she and Esther would have made together.

I keep getting flashes of this new yet familiar feeling — a feeling, not a thought; I feel it now — flashes — I don't know what it is; it is very pleasant and exciting; I keep thinking maybe it's autumn coming on, but it's something else. It doesn't seem to have a thought to correspond with it ... I think it might have something to do with Esther going to school — maybe I am catching some of what she is feeling; new teachers (a music teacher — I never had one of those); her kindergarten teacher, and another teacher for gym ... and Jodie and all the kids at the school bus stop at the bottom of Butterpot Road taking Esther under their wing ... new friends for her ... her world opening up.

... Yes, I think that's it; I'm catching (like a sniff of fresh mountain snow-wind) what she is feeling — the feeling of the big blossom of her world opening up; I feel as though it were mine.

Later: I can't help thinking there was something uncannily like my last sight of Granddad Hardy in that final glimpse of Jim: the hat; the way he was standing so straight and still, with a corona of aloneness about his ramrod straight body; straight and motionless — I was the one who possessed motion, and I was moving away from him, away from each of them: I was in a bus moving away from Granddad Hardy toward my tour of Europe. Today I closed the door behind me on Jim (standing there like that), moving toward the rest of my life ... Life.

September 16, 1994

I can hear the surf on the grey little beach breathing rhythmically beyond the inn window. Flowers are lone and sparse on a vast field which is all September sadness; fullness of summer, strawberries and gold warm light, all falling away to make room for frost and sleet and leaden clouds. A last spoonful of summer was the first evening here. I met Y on the sand — up to her knees in milky waves ... jellyfish all over the wet sand where the tide had gone out; milky warm wavelaps, golden rose sun setting, warm air and warm sea. I went in and got my scarlet rose swimsuit and plunged into the ocean, riding the swell and cutting through the crests.

Jim crying over the phone. Esther visited and cuddled into his back on the hospital bed. His hair shaved off now, that cap on. Tonight, crying, he said on the phone, "There's only one of me."

Wednesday, September 21, 1994

Just had a good conversation with Jim on the phone. Read to him John Donne's sonnet "Death"

> One short sleep past,
> we wake eternally,
> And death shall be no more:
> Death, thou shalt die!

He has been so full of grief and weeping, and missing Esther (though she has been in with me) — each time I see him now the rims of his eyes are wet, and he heaves great sobs.

Esther does not seem to get distressed, and goes up to him on the bed and holds him in her arms. She is strong, and comforts him by her love.

I felt good about tonight's call with Jim. I was able to tell him I love him, and I think he believed me.

Tomorrow the palliative care people are meeting with me, Jim and the social workers, to see if he is "ready" to go there.

He is not perceiving things the same way other people are; he is afraid. He wants to come home, and keeps saying, "If only this infection/cough would clear up, I'd be all right."

He asked me what I think of the palliative care idea. "I mean," he said, "the psychological thing — they don't try to make you better; they don't give you anything to try and cure you."

I told him I understood that he was feeling incredibly sad, especially over Esther. I said I could not enter into his suffering completely because I am not sick. I said I knew it must seem to him that I was able to do anything I wanted — go places, meet people, and that he couldn't. I said the Health Sciences hospital is ugly, cold and lonely. I told him everybody says that about it.

I told him they'd given him a death sentence anyway, he might as well spend the next while (always there is his hope he will get better) somewhere warm and comfortable.

Everyone says the palliative care unit is more comfortable and has a more caring atmosphere than the Health

Sciences. I told him the doctor said he could come home for visits from palliative care.

"How long?" Jim wanted to know.

"Overnight, I think," I said.

"That's hardly a visit," he said. "I want to come home."

I said the Health Sciences may "try to make you better" unlike palliative care, but they do it with a hands-off attitude, just administering pills and nothing else.

At least in palliative care they are present to really care about you, according to reports anyway. And no one can say you aren't going to walk out of there one day — it's been done before. No one knows for sure what is going to happen. You might as well spend whatever time you've got in hospital in a nice hospital.

This is what I said. (You can see from this what I want.)

"Are you starting to live without me already?" he asked when I was leaving earlier today.

He asked it again on the phone. I said, insofar as I was here, without him, trying to make a living and looking after Esther, with him gone, yes, I guessed I was. But he understood I needed to keep everything going, didn't he? I asked.

He said yes.

He said he is losing his mind in there — mainly out of boredom (out of grief too, I think) — He said he can't remember things such as our early days/years together, or who has been to visit, or what the doctors have said. He said his mother has noticed this. Is it true? he asked.

It seems to be. He always had an exceptionally good memory. Much better than mine.

Esther comforts him and loves him so very much. He lives on the love from her cuddles now.

Through Esther being in school, and through people's knowledge of Jim's sickness, neighbours are reaching out to us.

Thursday morning September 22, 1994

People say the wrong things to me. I realize more and more that only God and I know what is best for me. People say things like, "You should let him die at home," and, "You mustn't be too brave."

Let's take "You mustn't be too brave." (I believe we've already dealt with, "You should let him die at home.")

"You mustn't be too brave."

This was said to me in the hospital yesterday after I had seen Jim, by a kind and well-meaning woman. But there are things I know that she doesn't know: reasons why I must hang on to all my brave garments: my shield and buckler, my presence of mind, my undaunted faith in Christ's power, the sensible mind God gave me.

Reasons: — Esther: How would Esther feel if I crumbled and cried all the time?

— The bills I paid yesterday. I have to make payments on our life's externals.

— Myself: Yes, I can choose to enter into Jim's sorrow and dying and grief; but he has eternity at the end of his crumbling — I have "promises to keep, and miles to go before I sleep ...

... miles to go before I sleep."

... So, my kind L, you would like to see my sorrow, wipe my tears; maybe that's what would make you feel good — but right now I need to be a warrior: a brave warrior; and I am going to be that, with God's help. (Today our friend C told us that in Jesus we have "borrowed radiance.")

23 September, Autumn Begins 1994

Well, things are shifting around to a new reality.

Contradicting voices are beginning to merge.

I am beginning to see that I can bear only one course of action.

Today Esther surprised me by saying clearly (I have not discussed this name with her), "I hope Daddy doesn't have to go to the palliative care unit."

Across the round table in the kitchen, as we were eating noodles, tofu and shredded cabbage soup ...

"Why?"

"Because he wants home."

Now Jim is saying he cannot come home; we are not equipped, and he "can't function." I asked him how he would feel about my trying to get him into palliative care, and he said yes, do that.

Two women from there came to tell us about it yesterday.

Jim has been in the Health Sciences three weeks, and no doctor has touched him.

I am feeling relieved that:

(a) He is shifting toward accepting going there.

(b) The palliative women seem to be saying he would be accepted there if he felt ready to go.

I am feeling horrified and fearful that:

(a) There are no beds in palliative care just now.

(b) The social worker, helpful as she is, keeps talking about him coming home and trying to get me to believe it's easier to access palliative care "from the community" than it is from the hospital.

I am gaining determination through people like N, who is the only woman I know who has gone through what I am going through, and D, to stand firm and refuse to allow him to be sent home unless it is on leave from the palliative care unit.

N said: Tell them it's unacceptable for Esther to have this home situation.

D said: Get your family doctor to write a supportive letter saying you are unable to look after him at home in these crisis circumstances.

Conflict: Am I working my way out of what Jesus said to do?

Mother Theresa and all the saints? "She who seeks to save her life will lose it ... "

Left Hand: No. Jesus loves you. He is taking care of this. Don't waste any more of your beautiful life energy in this conflict.

I just wish Jim weren't so wretchedly miserable — if only

he was in palliative care now. Instead, he is going out of his mind in that cold, lifeless place.

Now that I have decided what my course of action must be, and now that he has moved to this position too, I can experience pure love, pure sadness for him (not warped by fear of having to cope with him plus all my other responsibilities). I asked him if he had any solace tonight and he said no.

What was it N said? She had such a beautiful and knowledgeable vocabulary for talking about all this —

Something like:

"It pushes you past the limits of what you thought you could tolerate ... " (meaning you realize you can't do it — can't do what they want — what you thought you would have wanted yourself to do.)

Why is it so hard?

W, whose husband has a degenerative illness, said immediately when I told her about the social worker, "They can't send him home. You can't be expected to do that. No one can do it, with a small child."

J said, "Would you visit me?" (in palliative care).

Please God let them get him in there immediately. So he can get some rest and warmth and comfort before he dies. God knows I never gave him any. (There is so much pain and fear — of him coming home — in my heart, mixed with sheer sadness for his sake because I do love him, that nothing I write seems to drain away the heartache.)

I'm going to have a cry ...

Song for Jim:

Every little thing
that makes life sweet
My daughter putting shoes
for kindergarten on her feet
Every little thing
that makes me smile
. . . is leaving me now
Every drop of rain
that wets the ground
or falls on my roof
with its comforting sound
Every drop of rain
I hear or see
may be the last rain for me
(and I don't know
I don't know
I don't know
how it came to this
and I don't see
I don't see
I don't see the Lord)
If you want to pray
for me now
these are the things
I want you to ask for
— all the little things
that make life sweet
— Let me hold them close to me once more

27 September 1994

Today they transferred Jim to the palliative care unit, which they call PCU.

Sunday, October 9, 1994

Before today Jim has always said, "If only I can get rid of this cough and get my strength back I'll be okay enough to come home."

Today he said, "I'm not getting any stronger. I can't get my strength back. The doctors knew it would be this way, didn't they, when they put me in here?"

He said, "I'm going to die, aren't I? Fade away — that's how it happens. Did the doctors disclose this to you? They knew, didn't they?"

I told him the doctors had told him the same things they had told me.

Until now it has always seemed (except during crises when he was obviously endangered) that he isn't really that sick — certainly not sick enough to die. Other people say, "Kathleen, he is very sick now." (Still, though, people are going in that room and dragging us by the hand into insensitive prayers that God will "shrivel up" the cancer etc ... also bottles of this and that "latest cancer cure." As he enters palliative care it seems people wielding these miracle prayers and shark oil cures have felt impelled to assault us with renewed vigour ...)

My mother said it is that way when someone is dying:

with her and her father she never did think he seemed sick enough to actually die.

To me it seems that he is still so powerful (except for today during his heartbroken/breaking realization) ... still has all the attributes that define him as himself.

My new friend L says it seemed that way exactly with her sister who died of cancer. "I never could believe she was actually sick enough to die. Her face was as pink and unlined as a baby's. One night she began to sing and sing. People in the family said that night that they believed she was getting better. She died within 24 hours."

Before now, Jim has, variously, talked of "coming home for Thanksgiving," "walking to get the strength back in my legs," (he has been walking regularly in the corridors, with his pale yellow wood cane, and his thin legs which he says are "like stilts." Now I don't know if he will have the heart to keep doing this, since his spoken thought today) ... and "getting Maud the occupational therapist to work with me on strengthening my legs." He said the latter just yesterday.

Also R came and prayed one of those awful "shrivel" prayers and I felt terrible and angry, especially when he and Jim together decided Jim had experienced "funny warm healing things" when R touched him. I could kill these people when they do this at this stage in things. Next time it happens I am going to interrupt them and make them ascertain what kind of prayer they expect from me; a shrivel prayer or a compassionate, real prayer that takes everyone's feelings (mine too) into account.

Tonight Esther and I had a lovely half hour cuddle/talk on the daybed in the kitchen before her bedtime. Esther prays her own things now. She prayed for Daddy to feel better.

Esther said, "If Daddy dies I will miss him so much. I won't be able to wait til I die so I can see him again."

I said, "We'll have to pray to Jesus to make us both strong enough to stand it, and to help us look after each other and care extra for each other."

After I said that she laid her hand on my heart and got me to lay mine on hers. Then she told me to close my eyes and she kissed my eyelids. Then I did that for her, and we held each other tight.

How's that for a beautiful, beautiful daughter?

The little mounds of her face are so mature — they are like the ancient globes of the sun: they are wise and childlike, knowing and pure, warm like tomatoes ripened slowly on the vine, in their own time: she is not like someone who is just a child: those warm, Aztec mounds on her face twinkle and dance like the starlit ocean in summer; warm, undulating, wise and deep; beautiful, embracing, and ancient and mythical. But still with the dimples of the illusion of childishness — the childishness that is knowing; the newborn-ness that is all-seeing; like the omnipotence of the child Jesus: the omnipotence not of the heart of him, but about him, like a cloak of star-dust.

I hope she is always like that, with her knowing, twinkling dimples and moon-mounds of her face.

What the palliative care unit is like:

1. Stained glass windows at the entrance and in the peaceful, quiet chapel; blue light and the beauty of holiness.

2. Caring nurses and beautiful doctors (women) who Jim says are like ministering angels. (There are only eight "beds" — rooms.)

3. Piano room, puzzles, toys, cartoons (Esther).

Beautiful food appetizingly arranged on pretty china dishes. Real cups.

5. Hand-crocheted coverlets.

6. Nurses that ask me how *I'm* doing, and who help me understand Jim's actions.

7. Other families/couches/coffee/fridge/microwave.

8. A spiritual component/resource library/inspirational and devotional books, tapes, videos.

What the other hospital was like:

—The cold waiting-room of hell. So pit-cold Jim always had wet eyelids from weeping.

—Curious note: Every other area of the hospital is well-signposted. There is no signpost pointing to the palliative care unit, which is along a red corridor and in an old, seemingly uninhabited wing of the hospital. Only when you are there is there a sign that says "palliative care," and the blue light, the beautiful stained glass window, and the sign that says, "Chapel: quiet."

It is as if nobody but the initiated are to know about this place's existence.

October 15, 1994

I feel like I'm not accomplishing anything. I'm raising Esther, doing the column, teaching my class ... but there are so many demands on me that are draining energy without giving me any reward or sense of accomplishment. I can't seem to think of what it is I really even want, except some love and warmth.

Last night, after Esther was asleep, I sat in the kitchen and sobbed out of loneliness — I was getting a taste of what it could be like here over the next fifteen years or however long it's just me and Esther here ... (of course I see when I write it down that that couldn't possibly go on that long, the same ...) — anyway, I was sobbing, and Esther quietly padded out in her jammies into the kitchen and started looking at me. She never does that: wake up forty-five minutes after she has fallen asleep. I said,

"It's all right, Mommy's okay. I'm just crying because I'm lonely."

She stood there by the woodstove looking at me.

"Did you come out to comfort me?"

"Yes — I heard you crying."

And she came over and got up with me and smoothed my face and held me in the warmest, fluffiest, jammiest, most loving and comforting hug. I thanked her.

Wednesday, October 19, 1994

Jim said, "Merry Christmas," tonight as Esther and I left his room.

October 20, 1994

Walked several miles through the woods with Esther (who did not get tired or cranky but was a wonderful companion). We found tent pegs in the fairy meadow.

I have been talking to our Creator as Great Spirit God: this feels good since at this time he *is* spirit and not dwelling in the flesh among us.

I went to a lonely bog near the blond swaying reed river alone this morning and raised my heart and pain alone to the Great Spirit. I believe he is the one who gave us the tent pegs. We have been wanting to make a tent, the most beautiful tent in the world. Esther believes the Great Spirit gave us the tent pegs too. She said, "He's the only one who knew we needed them." They are beautiful and strong and sturdy and long, and there are four of them.

On our walk Esther also found:

- animal holes in the moss with little eyes shining down in them and clusters of caramel mushrooms. (I want to learn the mushrooms to eat. I could call a naturalist group and join — Esther could come now.)
- two dead trees full of woodpecker holes. One had a really big hole. "That big hole is exciting," she said.
- moose nibbles (She nibbles too.) I saw today that when she is expressing something to me, she *enacts* everybody's and everything's part. She is waterfall and fox, rainbow and flames. We sat and rested at Bluehills View, and resolved not to do this again without bringing a snack and something to drink.

October 21, 1994

This morning Esther and I stole a look at the blue moon and frost-sparkling whitened marsh before the school bus.

Last night I found this quote from Emerson:

> "No change in circumstances
> can make up for a defect in character."

Here is the short dream I had just before waking this morning:

I am driving down a country road. Someone is in the car with me. I see a beautiful gray wild and free horse. It is running along meadows outside fences near the road. Too near the road. I turn away and all too quickly I am at a crossroads. There is a stop sign. I can't stop. I'll just have to go really fast through the crossroads, I tell myself, and hope nothing is coming from the right or the left. Actually nothing is, but that is not what I have to worry about. There is no continuance of the road straight ahead. There is just a cliff, over which I have just hurtled.

Saturday, October 22, 1994

At 6:15 am today Jim died.
The phone was unplugged.
Michael was called at 6 am.
He got there just 2 minutes after Jim had died.

Colleen came up to my bedroom on her way to the hospital with Gord, Bernice, Ryan and Vanessa and told me, at about 8:15 am.

I got dressed and dropped Esther off for a day of happiness with Jim and Barb and the kids. Jim is going to be one of the pallbearers.

I had been going to drop Esther there anyway: had intended to go and spend the day with Jim after Barb asked me to: she thought he was dying — would die soon. She offered to take Esther *last* night but I said no, today would be okay. She knew. The nurses didn't really know like Barb did, even though they were totally with it all through. I talked to one last night on the phone. He was asleep. I said tell him if he wakes up and you're still on that I'll be there in the morning. I don't know if he ever got told that. I do know he drank a bottle of Blue Star and ate a bologna sandwich last night. The nurses and I laughed over that. He never changed, they said.

I told Esther in her room. She cried. "Why couldn't you tell me later?" I said I was going to say goodbye to Daddy. It would just be his body. Did she want to do that too, or did she want to go play with Grayce and James, Alison and baby Robert. She said she wanted to say goodbye to Daddy's body at the funeral, and go play with her friends today.

"How long did he have, to say goodbye, Mommy?" she asked: "How long was he in the palliative care unit?"

Then she said, "Mommy, I'm glad Daddy had the long time he did have, to be with me."

I was surprised she thought of it that way. I said, "Me too, puss. And you know what? Daddy lived the long time he did so that he could be with you."

I spent some time with his cold body in the room alone. I

felt his spirit still lay enfolded, sleeping inside the dead body: it had not risen on its wings yet. I thought of Jesus' resurrection: the resurrection happened after three days.

I kissed his head. I placed a cross on his forehead with my finger and prayed that his spirit would be able to escape free into eternity. I pulled his sheet back and held his hand. That felt good. When I went to take away my hand it felt as if he clasped mine before he let it go.

It seemed his body was still rhythmically rocking, the way a dory seems to even when it is on the dry beach.

Esther is looking forward to the wake.

I had a private talk with Jim. It wasn't much. I asked him to forgive me. I said well you're dead all right.

I told Sharon he certainly looked dead. I never saw anybody look so dead. We laughed. Someone asked me if he just looked as if he was asleep. No. I said: he looks dead!

"He died with the falling of the leaves" (his mother).

Thursday, November 10, 1994

At six thirty on the second Saturday morning after Jim died I was woken by fluttering at the eaves over my bedroom window. There were two slender brown birds. They were a warm mahogany colour, and they were rustling and muttering peep peep peep. They were big, the size of jays, but more slender, much more graceful, with slender throats and bodies like plump young maidens. One flew into the trees and I saw that it had a beautiful fanned tail. They rustled about some more and I wondered at them: I had never seen such a bird before. Later in the day I saw, sitting on the scaffold that Jim's father had made years before he died, through the window beneath the one in my bedroom, one of these same birds. I could tell it by its beautiful slender body and its large size and its grace and its mahogany colour. But what I could now see, which I had not seen before, was that on the back of its head, down to its slender neck, was a beautiful ruby mark of an intense hue.

Tonight in my journal class I said, "Does anyone here know about different kinds of birds?"

L immediately asked, "Did you see a token after Jim died? I didn't like to ask. I made you a red bird for Esther."

H said the second day after her husband died, her son told her secretly at the funeral home that that morning their house had been the only one on the street covered with unusual white birds, so many that you couldn't get a pin between them.

J said that on the anniversary of her son's plane crash death, an unusual bird with red on the front of its throat woke her, singing over and over the name of one of the other young people killed.

L was given butterflies as tokens, and four purple fairy caps —her daughter's favourite colour, "and you never see purple fairy caps."

November 22, 1994

It's hard to assimilate any new information when there are so many "flashbacks" and deep feelings over Jim's death, over loneliness, over "charting my course." The last two mornings I woke up under the pain of loneliness like it used to be before I had anybody — before I had Jim or Esther: the same except this time after a few minutes of it Esther climbed upstairs and cuddled into bed with me. Thinking — you're not so strong, Kathleen, after all; so independent; so able to journey through the wilderness ...

Sorted out Jim's music yesterday — to keep/ give away/ keep for Esther: Tallis Scholars; Bach's Mass in B Minor; Handel's Messiah boxed sets, and, after talking with Barb, one Strawbs album — From the Witchwood — I read the lyrics and they were beautiful like he always said, but I never could listen to them.

Was going to give Tallis Scholars to someone but played a small piece and the beauty of the choir changed the room into heaven and I couldn't — more heavenly than when he was alive. His music meant so much to him that to hear even a strain of it in the room — well it *is* him; too hard to bear. So the dearest to his heart I will keep for Esther, and tell her, "this is the music your Daddy loved; these are the sounds that were closest to his heart."

12 December, 1994

Esther: Did your Mommy get sad like you are now?

K: No.

Esther: Well, she mustn't have lived. To live, you have to get sad sometimes.

On waking in the night and being unable to get back to sleep; toast: tea ...

The kitchen is warm, simple and clean at night — one a.m. — in the birch wood heat. A candle, a Christmas cactus blooming, two shining oranges in a blue clay bowl, wooden chairs with cushions on the seats, a box of cut splits. A china sugar bowl full of sugar cubes, a half-bottle of red wine.

I have let down the cream lace curtain upstairs over the juniper mountain star window — the scene was too harsh, after the killing sleet. Tonight, through folds of cream lace and roses, the snowy mountain, the interlaced trees, and the shed starlight were as in a far-away dream; veiled, illusory, and lovely: beneficent and soft.

A Christmas Card

December 1993

James Wade

December 24, 1993, the new hours ...

The festival of light is upon us ... or nearly so. The other day Kathleen and I went for a long walk in the woods — it was a warm day full of golden light. "There's something special about this day," she said. "What is it?"

"It's the winter solstice," I said.

"I knew it!" she said. "A special day."

The next day she found our tree abandoned in the road, not quite perfect enough for someone. Our tree.

It was brought home and put up. And we quite naturally have all the trappings of Saturnalia. Lights in the greenery, decorations and colour; thus we unconsciously coax the sun back. See, sun, here —here is one of your children: it couldn't have its greenery without you. Its photosynthesis. Is the word "photo" Greek for light? What's "synthesis" Greek for?

❖   ❖   ❖

This book is an informal Christmas card, which I've planned to write for some time. It's to whom it may concern, and it may concern many. It's to Esther, especially. And Kathleen, especially. It's a record of this Christmas 1993, memories of Christmases past and thoughts, perhaps, on those of future years.

I love Christmas — in a way it's a Christmas card to Christmas.

❖   ❖   ❖

I think I know why our first married Christmas (1988) was the best ever. There were a number of factors: Esther was pre-natal: a babe waxing big in the belly; we lived in that beautiful penthouse apartment — the Gothic cathedral loomed in front of our windows, with its rose window: the churchyard's leafless trees and the snow which fell steadily; the ship in the harbour with lights in the rigging; the wine and beer and music and food; the tree, that first incarnation of all our trees...

But what was special was that it was *our* Christmas. For the first time in my life it was mine. No overindulging, no drunkenness, no fighting, no being the recipient of someone else's Christmas. Ours.

❖   ❖   ❖

We try hard, and in a large measure succeed, to bring Christ into Christmas. The festival of light is really the light of Christ. His advent dispels all darkness...and the darkness has never put it out. The physical light of the pagan festival was only a type of the spiritual light of God.

❖   ❖   ❖

Christmas Eve

Today we went into town, after an urgent, packing morning. It threatened to storm: this morning's rainy weather turned frigid with high cold winds. On the way we thought of turning back but were glad we didn't. As it was, the storm missed us: it probably veered off to the southwest. But not before depositing a nice dusting — a Christmas veneer just in time.

Julia Pickard's was aglow with the fullness of Christmas

134

— smiles all around, pleasantries, an excellent repast of steak-pie, ham, potatoes and salad. Presents were exchanged.

Then it was on to Michael's for a five-minute visit, and away we went in fear of the storm. The last we saw of M. he was locked out in the wind-chill, sprinting around the house for access.

❖ ❖ ❖

Tonight — special preparations. K's fragrant cakes. Esther off to bed early, tired. But not before she sent a letter to Santa Claus soaring up the chimney. We're tired. I've been running on adrenalin all evening. Now it's the early hours of Christmas Day here in my lair. Some Christmas orchestral music is on low on CBC.

Esther asleep is so exquisite. It's then we look long and hard at her; it's then we're together (me and K) as no one else can be: in concert over her. When I see Esther sleeping I get an idea of what she'll look like when she's a grown up woman. Then all her defenses are down; then there's no ego. "That's something to remember in heaven," said Kathleen. "Esther asleep on Christmas Eve."

And of course I will.

❖ ❖ ❖

The creches are out all over the world, in the glow of votive candles. And the world stands still for a day, to remember His coming. Really, where is secular humanism on the 25th of December?

It's true what someone wrote in the Bible: "Every knee

shall bow in the name of Jesus. And all shall acknowledge that Jesus Christ is Lord, to the Glory of God the Father."

Boxing Day morning

Some quiet time by the fire on the morning after Christmas —Esther is watching her Barney video (clutching her Barney teddy) for the fifth or sixth time. K. still sleeping — a rare sleep-in. The tree is alight. Music on low.

Last night it snowed hard. We had quite an adventure navigating back from Conception. The car kept losing power; Butterpot hill was a toss-up. But we made it somehow — thump into our parking spot. There's shovelling to be done today.

Christmas Day was too full of everything to find time to write here. But I have a list of images and thoughts which may convey it:

Esther's wonderment on Christmas morning, her complete trust and faith in Santa, that he was able to do the unlikeliest thing to make her day special (like switching Daddy's Barney video and using lace for a tie from Mommy's sewing basket). As long as such belief exists in the hearts of small children, Santa *is* real. As it is, he's realer than a lot of things.

It brings back the long-lost memories of our own Christmas childhoods. God bless it.

K. made a huge completely natural wreath from spruce boughs, berries, twigs and moss. It was too big to fit hanging anywhere, so she laid it on the deep-freeze in the porch, leaning up against the wall. As good a place as any; it's a Christmas greeting, filling the porch with an evergreen fragrance.

The unearthly, cerebral music of Hildegard of Bingen filled the house a couple of times. It's quite excellent. In contrast K. had the Labradorians *Our Labrador* and Ron Hynes's *Cryer's Paradise*. We were amazingly diplomatic.

The turkey was luscious and fell off its frame in steaming dinner-plate loads of meat. Dressing, cranberry sauce (with Cape Shore berries). Vegetables. Wine. All given, K. observed, every morsel a gift from someone, and by extension, God.

I played the Pickwick Christmas LP as we ate — I should say as Christmas dinner exploded in gastronomical ecstasy on palates, an all-out dinner. The turkey was browned just right. The dressing was delicious. It swam in gravy. It was deftly washed down with Blue Nun. Lips smacked, teeth chomped, minds purred.

We visited family in Conception for a couple of hours in the evening. More food. Gord and Vince under the weather with heavy-duty tippling. I hope it comes as a revelation to Gord someday, the blessedness of a sober Christmas. Till then it's "befuddleness as usual."

Back home through the storm. Too stormy, I think, for Colleen to go by Marion's and tape "Scrooge" with Alistair Sim for me. Me and Esther watched some of it on her b and w TV in her room. Esther cuddled in with delicious shudders during the ghostly visitation scenes, and asked pertinent questions. "Did he (Marley) look like that when he was alive?"

"Is he (the Ghost of Xmas Past) a nice ghost or a yucky ghost?"

Later K. took out the photo albums and had a tearful catharsis. It's cleared the air. Especially poignant, she says this morning, was the one of me with the infant Esther, standing by the Cathedral with "a silly grin on my face." We didn't know then — we were innocent of what was in store. Oh well, and indeed we are still innocent of what's in store. The apostle Paul, quoting one of the prophets extends that thought to its ultimate conclusion: "Eye hath not seen, nor ear heard, nor has it entered into the heart of man what God has prepared for those that love Him."

I feel the Spirit as I write.

❖   ❖   ❖

27 Dec. the wee hours.

Christmas continues. Boxing Day was punctuated by visits, by us and to us. We walked briskly down to Gerry Squires's — there was something more Christmasy about walking, arriving with rosy cheeks, etc. K. carried Esther half-way: the wind was damp and cold; 10 cm of wet snow on the ground.

We didn't bring a wren but should have — "St. Stephen's Day she was lost in the firs." But there was no need of one, for Gail ("Rise up, young lady") more than accommodated us ("and give us a treat"). We were treated to nuts and butter-tarts, hand-dipped chocolates and cognac. I brought Hildegard of Bingen to play for G.S. — it puts me in quite a refined mood. Esther played with her gifts of play-dough. Kathleen and Gail talked birds and medicinal herbs in the kitchen. Me and Gerry talked music and literature in his studio.

His Xmas tree was a convoluted driftwood limb which hangs year-round above the fireplace. Today it was strung with coloured mini-lights and glass tree ornaments (they were tree shapes). On the mantle were two copper plates with the images etched thereon — a Holyrood cottage and the purple raven. They added to the Christmas ambience.

Later, at home, Mom and Colleen and Deidre arrived for their Christmas visit. Its main feature was the three mothers waltzing with their children to Emmy Lou Harris's *Child of Mine*. My waltzing with Mom caused peals of laughter from all hands.

27 Dec. late night

The third day of Christmas was a pleasant, homey one. The weather did marvels — changing from blizzard to flurries to sun by the half-hour. Snow danced and looped in the trees, filling the windows with a living Christmas landscape. Our fire crackled. Yet more turkey and hash got eaten.

Old friends came with children. Jim and Barb, Jamey, Gracie and Allison. They made it despite the weather. It's the first time I've seen them both at Christmas in many years.

I played Plankerdown and Red Island for Jim. We drank dark ale. Kathleen was the graceful hostess, whose hands procured and prepared. Barb was a happy recipient. The kids played.

Before he left Jim shovelled out my car for me. Evening had come on; there was a full moon over Butterpot Mountain and blowing snow in the starry wind.

If there was no Christmas it would be necessary to invent one (to paraphrase an oft-quoted saying, about God I think). One needs this rest. Days of good food, warm fires, doing nothing but pampering your old body. God knows, we do enough chasing after dollars, striving to make ends meet. In the old days in Newfoundland, people worked their finger to the bone, eking a living off the land. But come Christmas, they did no work at all — but spent the whole twelve days feasting, partying and mummering. They took their Christmas celebration quite seriously (so to speak). There's something that can be learned from that.

As long as I live I intend to celebrate the twelve Days — The Feast of the Epiphany (Twelfth Day) really is quite special. It was then Christ was revealed to the Gentiles — represented by the Three Wise Men — already his mission was seeing a measure of success.

The beautiful word "epiphany" has come into our language — meaning any spiritual or quasi-spiritual revelation. I always think of Joyce's *Portrait of the Artist as a Young Man*. (the sea-weed girl).

Before I forget, another memorable thing was K's reading today of "The Selfish Giant" to Esther and me. That beautiful story always fills me with awe. It has the Christ-child, and silver fruit, and a winter landscape. And the wounds of love.

The Christmas tree late at night; with no one up but me. I'm writing this by the tree's light. Sparkling strands of tinsel glisten and slowly move with currents of air. Green boughs, each needle delineated in coloured shadows glowing. The lights — multi-coloured and bright, soft white with a string of sapphire like a constellation. Strings of silver pearls drape branches. A great red ribbon bow stands out. And birds perch here and there, nesting, singing. Among them a partridge. There are apples, and Santas, musical instruments, snow-flakes and bells, a rhinestoned reindeer, a glass angel, a fan, tiny wooden Xmas figurines, wreaths, a one-eyed unicorn ... As well, there's Christmas art, small repros of angels and nativity scenes, a stained glass St. Nicholas ... Topping the tree are the doves from our wedding cake, still soaring, still swooping ... Blessing our tree with peace ...

Dec. 28

Snow continues to fill the picture postcard of Butterpot. It's a skin-deep wave of foam on the deck; every fir branch is laden deep. Tonight, after a day of snowing and blowing, the stars are out and the full moon rides high. The winter landscape is complete.

At midday we walked up toward the powerlines to K's first rabbit snare. The winter woods were beautiful. Snow thickly fell. It was all to much for little Es. She cried with the cold and had to be carried halfway back. Nina visited in the evening.

I went for another walk, down to the store — not trusting the one run with the plow and sander, with my virtually untried (in winter) pony. (I really must do something about this jumbled sentence structure). Visited Gerry again. We drank rum in the studio. Gail bathed the dogs. Then I walked back through the silver snowlight in the Christmas town to a sumptuous repast of lamb (fried with gravy and vegetables).

Dec. 29. a.m.

Some quiet time alone this morning. Esther watches the Umbrella Tree; K gone across the Witless Bay Barrens with Stan to deliver butter, then to town. I've desnowed the car and had her started. My "var" fire smells good. Hildegard's music uninterruptedly fills the house.

Outside it's sunny. Snow lies thickly everywhere, cladding every evergreen bough; the mountain is a serene white presence. We're in the grip of winter.

Last night on my walk I noticed Dunphy's Funeral Parlour was a house of strong contrast. The dwelling area was beautifully decorated with red and green lights — strings of mini-lights lacing the window, electric candles aglow, the whole bathed in soft floodlights. The business part of the building, really one half of it, was dark — not a bit of Christmas to enliven its dark purpose. Snow had drifted about, dusting the windows and giving an ice-house quality to it, as if to say "no spark of warmth can be found herein. Be gone, about your merriment and leave this place to its grim function." It was sort of eerie. I think if I owned such a place (God forbid) I'd at least have a string of lights. And what happens if there's a funeral at Christmas? Does not the Advent of Him who came to offer Eternal Life transcend mere death and all its trappings? A Christmas wake could be wonderful. Carol singing, decking the place with boughs of holly, good cheer. God Rest Ye Merry Gentlemen.

Dec. 30, evening

A buffeting winter storm — the second or third of the season already — appears to have passed with not too much damage. I made it home with Esther from daycare on the storm's skirts. I was bearing a ham, a gift from Gord.

This Christmas is marked by a death in my extended family, but not close enough to affect me personally. What it means is curtailed vacations for Marion and Bill, surprise arrivals of Cheryl and Peggy Ann and even little Marissa (whom we have not met). Family dreams of white hearses at weddings and ceremonies for still-borns.

This morning, on waking, I found the cold nipping my nose, and thought on the water. Sure enough, it was gone. We were pioneers for half the day — with suitably frayed nerves — melting snow in the kettle, getting water from the brook. I visited Mom in the afternoon for a couple of hours. The water blessedly came back.

Later at home I had a deep sleep on the futon, with the wild wind without. Late night listening to one of Michael's

143

eclectic tapes —Dylan, Cowboy Junkies, Cohen, Buffy St. Marie. Maybe I'll have a beer.

New Year's Eve/Day

Kathleen read Psalms 126 and 104 at midnight. So beautiful to hear the unadulterated word after everything else. They deserve being repeated:

> Psalm 126
> When the Lord turned again the captivity of Zion, we were like them that dream. Then was our mouth filled with laughter, and our tongue with singing; then said they among the heathen, The Lord hath done great things for them. The Lord hath done great things for us, whereof we are glad. Turn again our captivity, O Lord, as the streams in the south. They that sow in tears shall reap in joy. He that goeth forth and weepeth, bearing precious seed, shall doubtless come again with rejoicing, bringing his sheaves with him.—(KJV)

On New Year's Eve the storm again failed to find us. Me and Esther shovelled snow. Esther had a great time shovelling and sliding, ruddy-cheeked in her snowsuit. We ate baked ham for supper.

On an evening visit to Mannie Buchheit's he conjured up a ghost of Christmas past — the German Xmas tradition of Black Peter. A mummer type, black eyebrowed and mustachioed would arrive gregariously to inquire if the little ones had been good. Oh yes, the parents would assure him, they've been good. Mannie had been coaxed from behind his mother's skirts and bidden to enter the great sack Black Peter carried. It was suddenly hoisted, to the child's alarm — but he was let out at once with his prize, an orange (the first one he had ever seen). The appearance of Black Peter was a great incentive for young Germans to be good.

He spoke, too, of the candle-lighted tannenbaum and the Christmas Eve tradition of opening the presents. I had a drink of rum there.

Sunday morning 2nd Jan.

A little bit of Christmas was salvaged last night. Esther's defective Miracle on 34th Street I found worked fine starting about a third of the way through. I watched it in the wee hours; Esther now has it on for the second time this morning. But I still must bring it back.

It's a charming movie, a keepsake. There's something especially quaint about colourized versions — I have no qualms about them. I'm sure scrupulous tinkerers might even make efforts to find out what the original colours were. The movie is set in New York City in 1947, with its vintage cars, fashions, and mannerisms. Kriss Kringle, though, is quite the proper Englishman, sort of a universal character. Natalie Wood is the little girl. "Mr. Kringle *is* Santa Claus." May he give my little one many happy moments in her girlhood Christmases.

❖   ❖   ❖

Evening

A good day. It rained lots, taking with it the surplus snow. The deck boards are again visible; our wood has reappeared. Christmas is winding down; we're beginning to think about work again. Today K. wrote a number of short encyclopedia bits on plants. I read. Esther watched videos — she has discovered Birch Interval (it has an Esther and a "witch," vital ingredients). K. and E. walked out in the rain (it was Esther's idea) and came back thoroughly wet. We had delicious pea soup, made on the ham bone.

❖   ❖   ❖

The wee hours — Listening to Red Byrd and the Consort of Viols — Elizabethan Christmas Anthems. That one has certainly grown on me: I didn't think much of it three years ago. I've even begun to like viols.

Am starting to think positively again. Simonton's book *Getting Well Again* is a good read. I talked with Jim Wight on the phone. Me and K. had belly-laughs in the kitchen.

Esther woke up late at night with a pain in her leg. Poor little thing. We concluded they were growing pains, gave her Tempera, and covered her with Effie's quilt heated up on the stove. I told her she'd be bigger in the morning.

Big news of the day: Stan Tobin is getting us a calf, which he will raise for us ... Now to bed, to read and sleep the showery night ...

❖   ❖   ❖

3rd Jan.

A full day. I left early in deference to interminable visitors; went to Gerry's, where Squires was executing his first portrait of 1994, his first also as a non-smoker. An interesting experience, which I've seen before many times.

I stayed a couple of hours, till he lost the light; I watched him blocking in the painting — the model was Kyran Pittman daughter of poet Al Pittman. The face started ghostly to appear on the paper, the nose and eyes subtly delineated with the tip of the brush. Squires built up the texture of the paint, underpainting, trying to establish a mood of some sort. As usual he was accompanied by baroque. "There's a lot of Bach strokes in my work," he said.

At times he loses the face under a wash of light beige on white; but it reemerges, like a face submerged coming up for air. The brush pinks in the full lips, browns the eyebrows. A light colour highlights the side of the face, the hair. Squires moves from one area to another, fluctuating, brooding over the inchoate work.

By the time he stops for the day the portrait has begun to become a likeness: the hair is darkened, there's a flush to the cheeks, eye pupils are softly delineated, a single brush stroke has outlined the nose. "I like what we've got," says Gerry. "A good start."

❖ ❖ ❖

Later I went on a sentimental journey to Conception Hr. I wanted to see the c ribs in the church, but the building was locked. All I could see was a clump of evergreen in the window when I stood on tiptoe.

No luck finding the key at the Renewal Center, but the woman there gave me a tour of the place when I told her what I was doing. A rambling mansion it is, with hardwood and chandelier (those priests knew how to live.) No art, though, to speak of except for a smoky print of The Angelus. In the renovated attic I looked out the round window at a postcard of Conception's Church (from behind) with the harbour and hills. The woman told me to try my luck at the Convent.

Another first for me, but still no key. Sister Theresa let me in and I had to content myself with the little creche the Convent has: butterscotch figurines in a bird's-nest size stable, cupped around with mini-lights. I saw the chapel as well — the pres dieu facing each other, the old stained glass (erected in the memory of so and so): Gethsemane, St. Patrick, The Little Flower, etc. I told her I'd be back.

Then I went to the new graveyard, to check that out. One could hardly ask for a more dramatic or out-of-the-way place to be laid to rest. I had an epiphany there. The area is fringed with groves of evergreen; the soundtrack is wind soughing through their branches. To the left, as you stand facing the entrance, the land falls away to Colliers Bay with water visible. Straight ahead in the distance The Blue Hills were silhouetted against the sunset sky, with Bat's Hill on the right, and Avondale's hills on the left. The impression is one of expansiveness: you're high up, can see for miles, the concerns of the living are far away.

The graves were silent under snow — the couple of dozen or so who have passed on in the last six or eight years. I walked back through the old graveyard. It was a mistake: I sunk in the crusty snow, into goulds, tripping over graves, not finding the path. I was out of breath. And there was a distinct eeriness about it; it was starting to grow dark. I thought, "Get out of here — you'll be here long enough."

When I finally reached the gate I found I couldn't get out: it was frozen into hardened snow and ice, impossible to move. There was a high wire fence with barbs. To scale it would probably mean tearing my clothes. I was locked in! It grew darker.

There was nothing to do but go back. This time I skirted the fence, though it was hardly better going. But I was in luck — I came upon a rent in the wire and slipped through unscathed. Jurgen Gothe on my car radio was most welcome.

After supper and a nap at Mom's, I came home.

❖ ❖ ❖

4 Jan. morning

Some overflow thoughts from yesterday. The Irish nuns in the Convent yard lie under identical celtic crosses. They all died young: two were thirty-eight, one was forty, forty-six, fifty. Their names — Moore, Joy, Leamy I recall. From the old country, they lie facing the sea. I wondered about their lives, growing up in County Waterford, coming out to Newfoundland in the 1870s, teaching, dying young. "They fretted to death," my mother said. Now they lie close to the church wall, skeletons in habits, bone hands draped with rosaries, oblivious to perennial midnight masses just yards away, votive candles, fading light in stained glass on a winter afternoon.

5 Jan. Evening

A day of rain and fog. I was in town for the first time since Christmas Eve. Wilted Christmases for sale in shop windows — bins of decorations slashed, gold brocade angels still bravely putting on a show. For all intents and purposes it's still the festive season; most lights still burn brightly. Everyone — or nearly everyone — is anxious to let sober reality resume its sway. I had a bag of french fries and a coke — very unfestive — in a greasy spoon.

I went to the MUN Library. For the first time in a whole year I felt free just to browse, without having to squirrel information for a term paper. Perhaps, should summer find me healthy, I may look into Chaucer.

I took home an armload of books — a massive volume of Yeats's poems, also John Clare, letters and autobiography by John Ruskin, and a book called *The Life and Times of Ebenezer Scrooge*. Lots to read.

On the way home the car behaved most peculiarly — losing power and bucking. Water in the line? Who knows. I thought me and Esther would be stranded coming from daycare — the car died. But we managed to get going after a short prayer. We made it in fine form to the bottom of Butterpot; then she died once more. After more prayer and a couple of false starts she went, miraculously, all the way up.

She continues to be difficult tonight — losing power and farting. We'll see what tomorrow brings.

❖   ❖   ❖

6 Jan. Twelfth Day

Christmas ends with love in our family...and peace. Today was uneventful, cold and snowy; we were housebound because of the car. It's back now, fixed. Today K. worked on some drawings, I read, Esther did her darndest to play (sans daycare). She's a good player.

It's late evening now; I'm up alone. I'm gazing at the tree, its last night. It's served us well. Gifts still lie scattered about on the floor beneath, some from last year: Clara and the Nutcracker, Beatrix Potter's Nursery Rhymes, a real piggy bank.

Somehow I don't think it's ready to end yet. There's a postscript planned for tomorrow, if we ever make it to the crib. And perhaps the tree may yet shine.

But officially it's Twelfth Night. And now to sleep. Sleeping — "that knits up the ravelled sleeve of care" — puts an end to Christmas 1993.

❖   ❖   ❖

Jan. 7, Friday morning

Finally, the crib. I write this with nipped fingers in Conception's church. Esther stands gazing at the Nativity scene.

The stable has a dormer roof; it is suitably grayed and mottled. Through a back opening the painted backdrop has a

151

road (to Emmaus?) winding over hills; the Star floods the sky with light. Crowding around the sides of the building is a cluster of half a dozen spruce and fir trees — a beautiful rustic touch. The floor is in gray, creased cloth, for all the world like rock. Unfortunately someone had taken it in their head to paint the figures in flat colours, with no attention to detail. But we soon get used to it. Three epiphany kings bear their gifts. One shepherd still doffs his hat, a young sheep shyly peeps from between his legs. The ass and the cow gaze benignly on. The baby Jesus, blue-eyed and blond-haired, is oversized, as big as the rest of the figures. It seems fitting. Joseph's cupped hand is sans staff. Mary kneels with hands crossing her breast. A wonderful crib, fragrant of evergreen.

"Goodbye, Baby Jesus," said Esther as we left. "See you next Christmas."

❖   ❖   ❖

October 1994

In Peaceful Caring Universe
(PCU)

Oct. 1st, 1994

With a Fall day it's time to finally write down my thoughts. My memories of the last six weeks are too horrendous to recall — I throw them away. Begone! My writing seems so cramped; haven't held a pen in weeks. Hopefully it'll limber up. Doesn't even look like my handwriting.

Traffic sounds come in from Lemarchant Rd. The old windows are leaf-shaded. There's radiators and other old fashionedness. What a relief! If I'm to be here for a while (I'm afraid I might) I want the space to be simple and my own. I want bits of Newfoundland — the soil which is my essence. I want God here.

Blackwood's door poster is emblazoned like a pulsating icon across from my bed — a magnificent study of light and dark and tilting planes of light. J.C. Roy's little seascape sets it off. I love the yellow sky. That's all thus far. I have Handel's Messiah (Hallelujah Chorus as I write), and an assortment of other tapes. I should make a list of tapes and books I want.

I don't know quite what my body is telling me. Certainly I came to the hospital with every intention of going home again. It'll be four weeks tomorrow. I'm still quite weak. And this cough just won't give up. We hope.

Nice visits today. Barb and baby were like fresh breeze and blue sky. Phil Heath came at the same time — good combined visit. Phil stayed longer. Good fellowship — he read from Isaiah and prayed, says he gets a blessing from coming here — feels the Spirit. God bless him.

Just looking at the gentle picture of me I keep in my Bible

— thin and bearded, the student of literature. Me now — ugly, bald and puffed with vulture eyes. I can't help it and incredibly I don't really care. But I can safely say that in my life I've been almost as humbled as it's possible to get and still walk about and smile. So I'll sigh and hope I may live long enough to look normal again.

Ken Baikie came after supper. He seems in good spirits. He read some Isaiah to me as well. Is going to bring some medieval poetry next time.

I think this is enough diary for my first try. Till tomorrow.

❖ ❖ ❖

5 Oct.

This morning a radiant angel bestowed this book on me. Came from Hutton's. I feel sure the music notation on the cover must be Bach. Who else?

I'm here a week now. This is the first time I've ventured out in the armchair. Feels good despite the coughing. My writing seems to have improved. I'm doing well in spite of the adversity of boredom and virtual abandonment by those closest. God sends me friends. I have my art, which soothes the soul. I have my books. Boyd Chubbs, who's become a good friend, yesterday brought me *Beloved Prophet* — the love letters of Kahlil Gibran and Mary Haskell. Great book. Brian Griffin wants to bring along a VCR. Then I'll be all set.

Today I questioned my doctor about divine healing — surely she's seen it. She admitted she had, but acknowledged the mystery of it all. She didn't know. Yesterday that young

Jeremiah who came with Phil came for my healing. His eyes were burning. He was bursting with healing. I believed him. I believe still.

I fear Esther is growing farther away from me, which is perhaps not a bad thing, if I am to die. It's been weeks and weeks since she's had a daddy around the house. Minimal hospital contact. I miss her so. She's still my little girl no matter what.

Hair — the first intimation that my visage shall not always remain a desert vulture garden — appears to be returning. There's stubble on my face, up the sides. Head hair can't be much longer. That'll be a relief. I hate the dejected humbled look baldness gives. I wasn't meant for it.

However, these are mostly negative thoughts, not in keeping with a peaceful, caring universe.

My window is open a few inches. Balmy October wind. Outside sun-filtered leaves are tinged with gold. The pleasant sounds of civilization intrude on welcome ears. Choral music on my tape machine — Mozart.

❖   ❖   ❖

6 Oct.

Time to write again. Of what, I know not. Gray fall day. Some rain, with leaves turning. I'm listening to Josquin, Okenhem, etc. Mood music. Cough bothersome of late.

I was thinking of the Pinch School, specifically of the walk to and from there, still indelible after thirty years. The barren meadow, with each rock in place, each stunted tree.

157

Winds soughing. The dry-wet mud path through the woods, crisscrossed by roots, skirted with goulds and alders. It turns into a dryer more open way, with stones as hard as flint, blueberry bushes. Then comes the gap, which we scale. Then a luxuriant valley, hills on one side, great for Indian ambush in summer, sliding in winter. Best sliding around.

❖ ❖ ❖

Oct. 7.

A bath. Sister Ricardo is a volunteer nurse. She loves her job. This morning, and every morning, she will gladly bathe you. I've given in. Such luxuriance having your back soaped with warm water and cloth, under your arms. Then thoroughly dried with soft towel. I do my front. Pajama bottom is demurely dropped; I wrap a towel around my legs. Sr. R. kneels with her pan of water to do my legs and feet. Feet feel like they're on cloud nine. Soapy fingers squish between my toes. She dries them deftly. Then applies a cream and baby powder. What a blessed service!

The new cough medicine seems so far to be the best yet. I actually have some semblance of normality on the go. It feels restful.

❖ ❖ ❖

Sunny Saturday, warm. Trying to retain energy in a losing battle with cancer is no easy task. Must keep my thoughts trained somehow. It's all in God's hands. It is a hard battle. God knows I have the *will* to live.

There's so much left undone. So much life I haven't lived.

So many silences, contemplations, books unread, winds felt, stars gazed upon, writings written, smiles smiled. I need strength. I need positive energy, but I've lucked out in that category.

An image I have of the incarnate word is a pair of strong hands, calloused and creased, rising out of the earth, cupping clotted clay or roots. The dirt streams away in rivulets through the creased palms. The hands stand clean, radiant.

Jesus came from the earth in that he was the Son of Mary. As a prenatal baby he was nurtured on the fruits of Galilee. Thus he sprang from the soil, just as we all do. But by the Spirit he was one substance with the Father. True God of True God. Oh, inscrutable mystery! That we may share it. That we may be partakers of that same Spirit.

◆ ◆ ◆

The news on TV is absolutely alarming. Such a thin veneer of civilization covers us, one wonders why the Lord tarries. Unspeakable atrocities are the order of the day — genocides in Africa and Europe, disasters in which everyone dies, cult suicides, invasions filled with bloody violence, earthquakes, etc. etc. Still, switch the channel and everything is money-grubbing normality. But there is none righteous, no not one. Thank God for Vision TV. The Gospel is on the air.

❖ ❖ ❖

10 Oct.
Thanksgiving Day, 7:30 a.m. — I feel a good energy despite being awake a lot last night. Josquin on the tape (Tallis

Scholars) is soothing. It was the first one I bought back in 1987 (actually a birthday present). I remember it playing in my room on Colonial St. as I tried to talk the St. Thomas's church organist into playing at our wedding. I think it was what sold her.

If I'm not mistaken my writing seems to be coming back almost to normal. I feel several pluses this morning. Maybe the chemotherapy is finally fading completely. I must endeavour to be more active today, rather than just lying about. Though I don't have many options. I have my street clothes now.

❖ ❖ ❖

Joe Trahey for breakfast. Rough and ready "put her up" talk to go with bacon, eggs over easy, juice and toast. But Joe is a good soul.

Sunny warm morning. Even though my trousers were decidedly too small I have my shirt on and that makes a difference. I almost feel I have enough energy to flee this tower today, like the little lame prince.

Still bald in my reflection in the black TV screen. My consolation is feeling my face stubble, where its wiry new growth, and my mustache which is coming in.

Bless the Lord, oh my soul, this day, and let all that is within me Bless his Holy Name. Amen and Amen.

❖ ❖ ❖

Later — I fell down today for the first time. I was in the bathroom, aware always of my draining leg energy. Chris Wong was visiting: I told him I'd be there in a second. When I pushed open the stiff bathroom door my energy seemed to backfire and in a second I was on the floor, a bundle of broomstick legs; I hit my bald skull on the edge of the radiator.

Well the nurses heard and came a fluttering. It was quite the endeavour getting me off the floor and onto the bed. Quite the sobering experience. Now I must walk as if each step may bring disaster, and that's a drag.

The Greenes dropped by from academia — promises of rich books to read. Gavin brought Henry V. Seddy was by at suppertime. He questioned me about funeral arrangements. "Where do you want to be buried?" "Home," I said. "Where else?" I was nonchalant. Have to be. There's great comfort in the thought of being laid to rest in view of the hills and forests of one's native place. A blessedness and a peace. Ashes to ashes, dust to dust.